nic Attacks

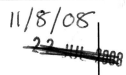

Panic Attacks

What they are,
why they happen
and what *you* can do about them

CHRISTINE INGHAM

Thorsons
An Imprint of HarperCollins*Publishers*
77–85 Fulham Palace Road,
Hammersmith, London W6 8JB

The website address is: www.thorsonselement.com

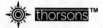

and *Thorsons* are registered trademarks of
HarperCollins*Publishers* Ltd

First published by Thorsons 1993
This updated edition 2000

9

A catalogue record of this book is available
from the British Library

ISBN 0-00-710690-4

Printed and bound in Great Britain by
Clays Ltd, St Ives plc

Contents

Acknowledgements

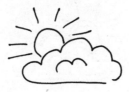

I would like to express my grateful thanks to all those who shared their very own personal experiences of panic attacks with me. Without them the book would be less than complete. Thank you.

Introduction

I know what panic attacks are like. I have experienced them myself, so I know how awful you feel when you have yours. I understand the fear you have about the next one. Like you, I've experienced the sheer terror an attack brings with it.

Some people have panic attacks on a daily basis; some are agoraphobic and know they would have them if they left the security of their home; others have them only infrequently when they encounter specific situations, such as flying or attending social functions. Occasionally, people may not identify what they experience as a panic attack at all. They may call it a funny turn, feeling peculiar, or going wobbly. Regardless of what you call it, if you experience feelings of panic, whether it's once an hour or once a year, this book is written for you. You may be male, female, black, white, old, young, British, American or from anywhere in the world. Panic attacks know few boundaries, and there are a huge number of people who have them. This book is for each and every one of you.

During the time I was having attacks, I know I would have appreciated a book of this sort. I wanted to find out all I could about them and what it was that was happening to me. Section 1 gives you this information. It covers the symptoms of panic attacks, why they happen, and the impact they can have on your life.

I also wanted to know what the possible solutions were. Section 2 deals with this. It looks at 'traditional' solutions and their strengths and weaknesses, based on current research findings. Complementary therapies are also discussed in this section. But the main emphasis is on healing the self, what that means, and how you can bring control back into your life.

One of the most important things I wanted to know at the time was what to do during an attack. They are so truly awful when they happen that I was tempted to think I would do anything to avoid another one. But attacks happen and I know it would have helped me build a sense of confidence if I had been aware of a few different strategies to employ in the event of another one. Section 3 looks at the possibilities. It also includes a chapter for friends and relatives. They can frequently feel at a loss as to what to do when you have an attack, so that chapter is written especially for them. The section also addresses panic attacks in children.

The aims of the book are many. The most fundamental is to bring a greater understanding through increasing your knowledge of what panic attacks are all about. Having such strong sensations wash over you without knowing why only adds to your fear. That fear can be much reduced through fully comprehending what is really happening to you – not what you *think* is happening. I hope the book manages to demystify the 'why' of panic attacks for you, and enable you to have a better insight into your own.

With this greater insight, knowledge and understanding I hope the book will enable you to realize how much you can do for yourself to bring your panic attacks to an end; there's a lot. I've included many suggestions drawn from examples of best practice which, without being prescriptive, will hopefully provide a springboard for your own thoughts and ideas to develop into your own personalized plan of action. You might like to have a note pad to hand to jot down not only notes, but also important thoughts which come to you while you progress through the book.

Another important aim of the book is to reassure. Because of the nature of panic attacks, it is easy to become incredibly fearful of them and to feel very alone in what you experience. The statistics will certainly show you are not alone, and the quotes from others who experience them will back that up. Reassurance that you will come to no harm is important, and I hope the book manages to provide enough of it.

You may be surprised by the fact that I look at the positive aspects of panic attacks. They do exist. Panic attacks can be a force for good. They have been in my life, and can be for you.

I realize that people who have panic attacks are often very sensitive people, and you may be tempted even now to put the book aside, not wanting to read anything about panic attacks for fear of bringing one on. I understand that. However, I would encourage you to continue. Chapter 1 is brief but important. You will see from it that panic attacks can and do come to an end; hopefully, it inspires you to read on. As you do so, you will soon come to realize what you can do about your panic attacks. Indeed, you have already made progress simply by opening this book.

Above all, I hope you enjoy reading the book as well as finding it useful. It won't in itself bring your panic attacks to an end, but it might give you some very positive ideas about how *you* can.

Section 1

Putting Panic into the Past

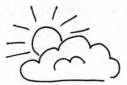

My first panic attack was devastating. The second, terrifying. In the wake of many others, I frightened myself even more by wondering if they would ever stop. To me, it seemed as if they never would. I began to think I'd never have a day free from worrying about them, and when the next one might happen.

When you have panic attacks you gradually begin to tiptoe through each hour, every day, wary lest you disturb that sleeping monster and nudge it into life again; the one which makes you quake with fear and trembling in front of its gnashing and awful jaws.

But be reassured, panic attacks do go away; they do end.

You find that hard to believe? Perhaps you do at the present moment, and if someone had said that to me a few years ago, I too would have doubted. So intrusive, debilitating and frightening are the attacks that it seems that all one does is wait warily for the next one, which you hope and pray won't happen, but which inevitably does.

No one told me that they eventually go away when I first started having them. I had to find out the hard way by living in that fearsome place next to the 'monster' for what seemed like an awfully long time until I too became free from them. During that time, if someone had simply reassured me that they wouldn't go on forever it would have given me a much-needed ray of hope. So by way of reassurance to you, here are some comments from people who, at one time, also despaired about ever being free from them, but who now are.

Karen is now 26, single and self-employed with a confident, chatty, bubbly personality. A few years ago, at a time when she should have been enjoying life to the full, she began to experience panic attacks over a number of months. After their repeated occurrence she too 'was scared they wouldn't stop' and began to wonder if she would have to deal with them for the rest of her life; it certainly feels that way when they recur time after time. They affected her so badly that she began to feel useless and as though she would never be able to cope with anything again.

Now, after overcoming them with the help of complementary therapies, she sees them in a very different light. Instead of something to remember with fear, she now looks back and welcomes her experience of them because 'It helped me understand myself better.'

Karen is now confident and happy. She leads a panic-free life and values what she has learned about herself during the time she experienced them.

Brian is almost the same age as Karen, in his late twenties. He's a design engineer and first began to experience his panic attacks when he was just twelve, and in the naiveté of youth 'assumed that everyone experienced them to a certain degree'. Unlike Karen, he used medication from his doctor to help stop his attacks.

Now, after having left them behind, he has used the opportunity which his experience gave him to identify factors in his upbringing and in his present lifestyle which may have contributed to the attacks. He has addressed those factors and as a result has resolved a number of important issues.

Brian is now free from panic attacks.

A similar raising of awareness happened as a result of **Jenny** experiencing her panic attacks. She was married and in her early twenties when she had her first one. They continued for about a year. The panic attacks coincided with money worries, concern over the vagaries of her husband's self-employment. and the additional responsibilities she carried in her job as a supervisor.

After experiencing her first attack she went to see her doctor who, fortunately, was sympathetic and knew something about them. He taught her ways in which to handle the attacks without medication. He also took the trouble to explain to her what they were. In finding out more about them she says that she then 'learned to deal with them better due to more of an understanding of them'. Knowing all you can about what it is you're experiencing is vitally important if you are to learn how to take control over them.

Like the others, she has found that understanding herself better has been one of the positive spin-offs from passing through this painful episode. It also improved the general quality of her life, bringing her closer to her husband. If it hadn't been for the panic attacks she may never have made these improvements – or even realized they needed to be made.

Jenny is now free from panic attacks and is 'confident enough for me to say that I doubt I'll have any more'. Perhaps that's how you want to be able to feel.

Colin experienced his panic attacks for a long three and a half years. They affected his life 'very badly indeed, making things impossible'. Unfortunately his doctor was unsupportive and did 'very little' to help apart from writing prescriptions. Eventually, dissatisfied with the treatment he was receiving and realizing he had had enough of the debilitating attacks, he decided to take control and sought help through a psychiatrist. There, at last, he began to make progress. Encouraged, he helped himself further by starting to make other very real changes to his life.

Through experiencing his panic attacks he has gained a new and better perspective on his life; he's made it much fuller and happier, making sure he includes more of the things he enjoys.

Like these people, I too look back on having experienced panic attacks in a positive light, although that wasn't how I felt at the time. I was confused by what was happening – and frightened. After the second attack I went to see my doctor who, like Jenny's, was sympathetic and understanding. She took the time to explain to me exactly what was happening. Medication was prescribed, but I confess I largely ignored it. Instead, I sat down to think. I decided that whatever the panic attacks were, they were certainly telling me that something wasn't right in my life. I couldn't see how treating the symptoms with a pill was going to help me uncover and treat what was causing the attacks. Only I could do that.

Looking back at the time when they began, I'm now only surprised that I didn't have one sooner. But I'm really thankful that I eventually did. Yes, you read that right, I am thankful. Although I wouldn't wish them on anyone, I understand and appreciate the ultimate benefits they can bring – if you choose to look for them. For me they proved to be a turning point in my life which was, at the time, giving me little satisfaction. I also realize now just how lacking in awareness of my body and my self I really was. The panic attacks were my subconscious telling me that all was not well with my life. They were trying to wake me up to a few rather uncomfortable truths. Panic attacks can serve a useful purpose.

But now for many years I too have been free from panic attacks. I state that proudly; not to gloat over those of you who have yet to put them behind you, but to encourage you, to help you see that distressing though they are, they do end. Whether you have had them for just a few months like Karen, or for years like Brian, you have the opportunity to turn this experience into something positive for you and to start putting them behind you. The people I have briefly mentioned have all gained to a greater or lesser degree from having had panic attacks. As you progress through the book I hope you too will find ways in which you can start to turn this difficult phase in your life to your advantage, as well as taking reassurance from the knowledge that you are not alone in what you experience, that you will come to no real harm when you have one, and that they can, and do, eventually end. Does that make you feel better already? I hope so.

Let's start by taking a good long look at this 'monster'; staring it straight in the eye, and demystifying what happens to you during an attack. Prior knowledge and understanding can help take the fear away about what is happening or what you think might happen. Then no matter how big the monster is, if you have no fear of it, it simply doesn't matter at all.

Summary

◆ Panic attacks can, and do, come to an end. They have for others, so why shouldn't they for you?

◆ Panic attacks are unpleasant, but they can serve a useful purpose in your life – if you choose to see them in that way.

◆ You are not alone in what you experience.

◆ Knowledge and understanding are important in helping you gain control over them.

◆ You are already making progress towards living a panic-free life by deciding to read this book.

2

Anatomy of Attacks

Although there appears to be a lack of awareness among the general public about panic attacks, the medical profession have known about them for at least 90 years. At the turn of the century, if you experienced them you would be variously diagnosed as having neurasthenia, irritable heart, anxiety neurosis, or DaCosta's syndrome, named after the doctor who noticed its common occurrence in front-line soldiers. But it wasn't until as recently as 1980 that panic disorder was recognized as something quite separate from general anxiety and given its own list of diagnostic criteria to help doctors identify it in patients. Perhaps its relatively recent appearance on the medical scene explains the lack of both public and professional awareness, as well as the dearth of literature available for the layperson. And in order to learn how to deal with panic attacks and take an active part in your own healing process, you do need information. So let's start with some facts.

How Common Are Panic Attacks?

Panic attacks have been identified the world over. Many studies have been carried out to ascertain the number of people who experience them, and the results show that between one and two per cent of the population have panic attacks on a regular basis, i.e. at least four attacks in a four-week period. Around 10 per cent of the population have intermittent panic attacks, and one extensive study in the USA revealed that a startling 35 per cent of people have had at least one panic attack – a staggering 87 million Americans. Small wonder that D A Katerndahl at the University of Texas noted that 'there is increasing evidence that panic disorder is a major health problem in the United States.' And if these figures hold true for other countries this means that, for example, in the UK over 20 million people may have had at least one panic attack, and nearly 9 million in Australia.

Based on these figures, the chances are that every time you sit on a bus with twenty people, seven of them could have experienced a panic attack. Knowing this makes it understandable why panic disorder is noted as being the most common anxiety problem for which people go to seek help. So you certainly need not feel alone in what you experience, and you can take comfort in knowing that many, many others are in the same position as yourself.

When Do They Begin and Who Has Them?

Most people have their first attack when they are adolescents or in their early twenties. Apparently it is rare for them to begin past the age of forty, although people can continue to experience them beyond that age. One study of children who were being seen for psychiatric help with specific problems revealed that a considerable number of them (26 per cent) also had panic attacks. The youngest were only four years old! So although attacks begin for most people between the ages of 15 and 40, even little children can have them.

In terms of differences between the sexes, some clinical trials appear to suggest that it is as common for men to experience them as women, but other studies suggest that more women than men have them. Many factors come into play as to when, why and to whom they occur. It's a complex picture and will be dealt with in more detail in chapter 4, but in general, it's been suggested that people who panic tend to show a high degree of conformity: always doing what they're told and what's expected of them. But that really is only one element; there are many more to consider, some of which are discussed later on.

The First Attack

Many people's first attack tends to follow the same pattern. You will be doing something quite ordinary like reading, driving, watching television or eating out when . . . *zap*! Before you know what is happening, you find yourself in the middle of your first panic attack. In my case I had had a relaxing evening at home and had gone to bed early after a long, hot bath, taking a new book with me. I was totally engrossed in 'whodunit', when suddenly, there I was having what turned out to be the first of many attacks. To say I was surprised would be an understatement.

Some people have their first attack while they are asleep and find themselves abruptly shocked into waking, but not because of a bad dream. Instead, they will have been sleeping quietly when suddenly it strikes; this must be very disconcerting.

Most people have their first panic attack spontaneously, apparently with no prior warning; but some do have them during a particularly stressful moment, such as when they are giving a talk to a group of people, taking an exam, or attending an important meeting in which they have to take an active part.

No matter where or when they start, there is a great deal of similarity in the symptoms people have. Whatever you experienced in yours, you can be reassured that others will also have felt the same. 'What, really?' you might ask in a doubtful tone. The answer is a resounding 'Yes'.

Symptoms

There are a number of symptoms which you may have experienced not only during your first, but also during subsequent attacks. See if any of these sound familiar:

'My body froze like a statue. My pulse would race very, very fast. My sense of reasoning and perception would become completely muddled and confused.'

'Terrifying.'

'A ringing in my ears would occur and my body temperature dropped.'

'It happens very suddenly – I feel faint, hot and sweaty. My heart beats rapidly. I feel I can't move or speak and that I just want to lie down. My stomach and chest are churning inside.'

'Numbness in my hands and then this feeling that I couldn't breathe. A feeling I was going to have a heart attack and a dryness in the mouth. Hearing my heart going; palpitations and an overwhelming fear that I was going to have a heart attack and die.'

'A tingling sensation down my left arm. A constant pain above my chest; also tightness of the chest. A cold sweat. The need to breathe in more air. Total panic and shakes. I had thoughts of fear that it was a heart attack.'

And Brian listed his symptoms as: 'High heart rate; sweating; flushing sensation in head; twitching muscles; feeling of coldness in hands and feet; wanting to go to the toilet. I thought I would collapse or faint, or even die.'

My own experience with my first attack when I was comfortably reading my book in bed, was that first of all I started shaking quite violently and then sweating profusely. I remember noticing I was breathing heavily and then I had an overwhelming desire to go to the toilet, and very quickly had to dash there. A feeling of terror started to overwhelm me; during later attacks the terror took the form of thoughts that I was either going to die or lose my grip and go mad. Of course I didn't, and haven't since. Neither has anyone else. Neither will you. But the feelings you have are incredibly unpleasant to say the least, and the full horror is difficult to convey to someone who has never experienced them. One analogy I read likened it to suddenly finding yourself looking into the jaws of death and experiencing the full terrifying horror of what you might see there. Yes, I think that's a fair description of what mine felt like.

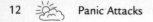

The *Diagnostic and Statistical Manual III Revised Edition* (DSM-III-R) lists the full range of physical symptoms which people may experience during a panic attack. These are:

- shortness of breath
- fast heart rate or palpitations
- pains or discomfort in the chest
- feeling smothered or as though you are choking
- feeling faint, dizzy or unsteady
- feelings of unreality (depersonalization and derealization; discussed below)
- tingling in the extremities, or numbness
- hot and/or cold flushes
- sweating
- trembling muscles or shaking
- feeling nauseous
- wanting to go to the toilet.

You probably won't experience all these things at the same time. Apparently, people on average tend to report having about seven different symptoms.

Besides the physical sensations, people tend to share similar thoughts and feelings too. These are:

- a sudden overwhelming feeling of fear, terror or apprehension
- an awful sense of impending doom
- being frightened you might die
- being scared you might go crazy or lose your mind
- fearing you might lose control completely.

Although terrifying, none of these thoughts and feelings ever comes to anything. There is no evidence that anyone has ever died from a panic attack, and no one has ever gone crazy. Neither has anyone completely lost control of him- or herself. *There is no evidence of anything bad ever happening to anyone during a panic attack, no matter how frightened they have felt.* So be reassured that although what you feel is extremely unpleasant, you will come to no harm. It's important that you realize this, and I'll keep reminding you of it throughout the book.

There is one particular combination of symptoms which is quite common and worth mentioning: palpitations, sweating, shortness of breath and a fear that you might be dying. It's important only because those who have this combination tend to think they're having a heart attack, like a few of the people quoted above. Typically, they may rush themselves to hospital, fearing the worst, only to find that the doctors pronounce their heart is strong and sound. Although people obviously feel a great deal of relief in being told that, they can also leave the hospital feeling confused and still somewhat frightened if the doctor doesn't reassure them enough. They know they felt something powerful, very real and frightening, and without a proper explanation they may still harbour fears that they haven't been told the truth, or that perhaps next time it will be a real heart attack.

Another common feature of panic attacks is how they appear to strike 'out of the blue' and without provocation. This makes them markedly different from phobic reactions which are provoked only in response to specific feared situations or objects. However, having said that, people who panic can eventually come to identify panicking with, for example, driving a car or going to the supermarket or any other situation where panic attacks have occurred in the past. In this way some people might become agoraphobic. Not knowing when another attack might happen creates another fear in itself on top of the one you already have about panic attacks. You're scared and on edge, fearing the unpredictability and wondering where you might be the next time, and it is all too easy to assume that you will again have one in the same place or situation where you experienced one in the past. This not knowing creates another fear in itself on top of the one you already have about them. You're scared because you're never quite sure just when another attack might happen, or even if it will happen at all. It keeps you on edge, fearing the unpredictability, wondering where you might be next time.

Development of Attacks

Most attacks last for between 5 and 20 minutes, although they can be as brief as a few seconds. Some people report them lasting for up to an hour, but this is very rare. What people might be experiencing is a wave of one attack after another, or they may confuse a feeling of continued anxiety or agitation with the initial attack. However long yours last, they probably leave you feeling rather jittery, ill at ease and also quite exhausted.

The number of attacks and the frequency varies from person to person. A lot of people have just one or two attacks and no more, while others have several in a week or even in a day. Mine, for example, happened every other week or so and were limited to a relatively brief period of about six months with just one recurrence some time afterwards. Others, like Brian in chapter 1, have attacks for years before finding a treatment which helps send them into full remission.

There tends to be no regularity to the pattern of attacks; in fact, their irregularity is one of their features. It's not like having a toothache which is exacerbated by eating ice-cream. How often they strike for you will depend partly on how anxious you are in general, but you might like to start keeping a note of just how many you have; the time of day; where you were and what you were doing. You might find you have far fewer than you imagined.

Panic Disorder

Not all people who have panic attacks can be said to have what is called panic disorder, as classified in DSM-III-R. You only have it if the attacks are particularly regular and frequent. You must have had at least four panic attacks in a four-week period. They must have been spontaneous and separate from each other. Or, if after one attack there is then a significantly high level of anxiety for at least a month afterwards about having the next one, this also meets the criteria for panic disorder. DSM-III-R also specifies that at least four of the symptoms listed above must have occurred during at least one of the attacks, for them to be classified in this way.

This book is for anyone who has had a panic attack, regardless of whether they have been told by their doctor that they have panic disorder or not. But it's important that you know what is meant by the term, to avoid confusion when it is referred to later on. Whether the doctors want to give you the label of panic disorder or just simple panic attacks is up to them. What's important for you is to understand as much as you can about what you experience, and find ways in which to move towards a panic-free life.

The Fight or Flight Response

One of the main symptoms of panic attacks is an overwhelming feeling of terror and physical fright; a very similar effect is produced by the **fight or flight response**.

This is common to all animals, including humans, and normally comes into play only when the animal is faced with danger. When we are, it takes a split second for the body to prepare itself, assess the possible outcome and take action. If it looks like we can overcome the danger or confrontation and win, the action we take is to fight. If, however, our quick-fire assessment shows that we would be likely to lose if we did stay to fight, our body is equally prepared for taking flight and running away from the threat. This is all done automatically; we don't have to think consciously about doing it, in the same way we don't have to think about making our heart beat. It's handled by the autonomic nervous system, which is entirely separate from the skeletal nervous system whose nerve endings respond only to direct physical stimulation and which, for example, pulls our hand away from a hot flame.

So let's assume you have suddenly found yourself face to face with a roaring lion. What happens?

Firstly, the senses send messages to the outermost surface of the brain about what they note has just happened, i.e. 'There's a whopping great hungry lion here!' The information is combined with all our memory files to compare notes. Lo and behold, the memory comes up with a match with something it vaguely recognizes, and wisely concludes 'This means danger!'

At this point a message is sent deeper into the brain to what has been identified by scientists as the primitive centre; it's called the hypothalamus. Its function is to coordinate all the activities of the body which are not in our conscious control, such as heart beat and metabolism. It is situated just above the pituitary gland.

Once the hypothalamus has received this message that all is not well, it raises the alarm and calls on the pituitary gland. This is the gland which controls and governs our endocrine (hormone) system. Once alerted, it produces a hormone which activates the adrenal glands. They're found just on top of the kidneys. When the adrenals receive the alert they produce adrenalin (epinephrine) and noradrenalin (norepinephrine) – hormones which prepare the body for action; for fight or flight.

The effect of these hormones is immediate and drastic. This is what happens:

◆ The liver releases its store of blood sugar to send to muscles for quick energy.
◆ Breathing becomes faster to take in more oxygen. Oxygen is needed by muscles to help transform sugar into energy. Faster breathing also helps get rid of excess carbon dioxide.
◆ The heart beats faster to transport the oxygen-carrying blood to the parts which need it in time. As a result of this increase in heart rate, blood pressure rises.
◆ To conserve energy there is a shutdown of non-essential operations like digestion. Secretions also stop, so for example the mouth is left feeling dry.
◆ The bladder and bowels may evacuate any excess loads they are carrying.
◆ Sweating increases in order to cool down the skin which, during the imminent action, would become hot from the body's exertions.

- The senses become more alert. The slightest touch provokes a reaction; sight and hearing are enhanced; you may 'smell' fear.
- Blood is diverted to muscles away from areas which don't really need it, so you may become pale.
- Tensed muscles give off lactic acid into the bloodstream, which has the effect of increasing anxiety.

Believe it or not, this comprehensive list of actions all occurs in just a matter of seconds. We don't even have to think about doing it – it all happens automatically. It's worth remembering too that this adrenalin release, and its subsequent effects on the body, can happen in moments of pleasurable excitement, as well. So although we have talked about danger provoking its release, excitement of any sort can. You will see later that this may be of some significance to you.

Looking back to the list of panic attack symptoms, you can see the similarity with the fight or flight ones. Even the heightening of our senses may be significant, perhaps accounting for why brightly-lit supermarkets can be a difficult place for people who panic to cope with, causing their already heightened senses to become overloaded and as a result create feelings of stress and anxiety.

Understanding this similarity helps it all to make a bit more sense. The reason why you experience the things you do is simply because your body has tripped the adrenalin release switch and started to prepare your body to either fight or run away from the lion it thinks it has seen. This is what Melanie experienced very clearly in her panic attacks and said 'You can feel the fear but it feels like a chemical going all through the body'. That's exactly what it is. What you experience in a panic attack is a basic and natural response to a danger signal which the primitive part of your brain, the hypothalamus, has given. The symptoms are the result of a life-saving mechanism springing into action. You have nothing to fear from them, in fact quite the contrary; your body appears to be trying to protect itself and save you from harm. Think about this because it may help you start to think of them in a very different way. They're not there to harm, but to help.

Derealization and Depersonalization

Feelings of unreality are common either prior to having your first attack, during one, or in between them. It can be an unsettling experience. Melanie tried to describe some feelings which she'd experienced and hadn't understood like this: 'seeing the reality of life and yet not being there . . . a Disneyworld dream state . . . it's as if the normal life we live isn't really real.'

These feelings of unreality are described as either depersonalization or derealization. To distinguish between the two, depersonalization is when you have a feeling that you are somehow detached from your body; as though you are floating some way above or just outside yourself. Derealization is apparently more common and is when you are grounded in yourself, but you can't quite find your place in relation to things around you. You might even feel unsteady on your feet. From Melanie's description, it seems as if what she was experiencing were feelings of depersonalization, and not the more common derealization.

Although these feelings are very disturbing, they too are protective mechanisms. Isaac Marks, researching into this phenomena, has suggested that the mechanism comes into operation when your feelings of anxiety have reached too high a level. Other research suggests that during these feelings of unreality, your anxiety levels actually drop significantly. So if you experience feelings of either depersonalization or derealization, you should be quite pleased with yourself! Your body is acting on your behalf to save you the unpleasantness of experiencing any more anxiety. There is nothing to fear from the feelings, especially now that you know what they are and what they are there for. In fact you could start to welcome them, now that you know they only happen as a way of helping you to cope.

I hope that this explanation of what is going on during an attack has given you a greater understanding of what is happening to your body, so that you can begin to feel more calm and less fearful. The quaking, trembling and other sensations will still feel unpleasant, but now you know *why* your body is doing that, it should help take some of the fear out of the attack.

In the next chapter, we can go on to consider the broader impact panic attacks can have on your life.

Summary

◆ There are an awful lot of people who experience panic attacks. You are not on your own.

◆ Although the feelings you experience are incredibly unpleasant, they will do you no harm. You will not die, go mad or lose control; neither will you have a heart attack.

◆ The sensations you have are all because you have suddenly had a large amount of adrenalin released into your system.

◆ Adrenalin is a way of preparing your body to protect itself. Ask yourself: what is there to fear about being protected?

◆ Depersonalization and derealization are also mechanisms which act to protect you from feeling any more anxiety. Try to welcome them next time; they're actually doing you a favour.

3

The Impact on Your Life

A lot of people who experience panic attacks avoid seeking treatment or help from their doctors. There may be many reasons for this. Perhaps they think they would have an unsympathetic hearing, or that their misplaced fear of being told they are crazy or mad would be realized. There may also be an unwillingness to accept fully the existence of attacks even to themselves, let alone others. It can take a lot of courage to tell someone the way you feel. It's not as easy as saying you have a sore throat or a broken leg.

If you are reading this, you have acknowledged your attacks, to yourself at least, and are curious to know more about them and what you can do to bring them to an end. By deciding to read this book you've made a step forward already.

I have mentioned the need for you to have as much information as possible about panic attacks. By knowing the facts, you can start to remove the fear which surrounds them. Now we can turn to the reasons why they have had such an impact on your life. It should help you get them into proper perspective.

Sensitization

Your first attack was probably extremely unpleasant, and to some extent shocked you. 'Where did those sensations and feelings come from?' you might have wondered. Because the experience hit you with such force, and so unexpectedly, it probably had the immediate effect of conditioning you into fearing the next one and when it might happen. At that stage, the only thing you did know with any certainty was that it was horrible, unpredictable, spontaneous and you didn't want another one.

This fear of the next attack can have a profound effect on your life. On top of the usual day-to-day worries you now have this other, very potent fear: that of the next attack. Fear is an incredibly strong emotion. It has the effect of priming the autonomic fight or flight response, which was discussed in the last chapter, into readiness. As a result you begin to feel on a knife edge without knowing why. You suddenly find that you can be roused with alarming swiftness. You may lose your temper too quickly or find yourself feeling frustrated much more easily than you used to. This state of arousal has been called sensitization.

So instead of calmly going about your day-to-day activities, and taking things in your stride, you find your emotions becoming worn out simply because they have become exaggerated in this sensitized state. Melanie told me she felt 'totally debilitated' during the time she had her attacks. You may find yourself more nervous and apprehensive, and not just because of worrying about when the next attack might be. There is a definite feeling of general unease. And because you haven't had the attacks properly explained to you, the bewilderment and fear you already have about them is probably increased even more.

In feeling bewildered it is easy to understand such thoughts arising as 'Am I going crazy?' or 'Am I losing my mind?' No, you are not going crazy or losing your mind. All that has happened is that you have become hypersensitive. That doesn't constitute madness in anyone's book. Hopefully, now you understand why you may have felt a sense of confusion, you realize that you are perfectly sane and will remain so. No one who has panic attacks has ever lost their mind or gone crazy because of them. There is no research which has found any such thing happening to anyone.

Being in such an anxious state, which you may not be fully aware of, you may find daily activities affected. Your concentration goes and decision making becomes more difficult. 'Should I have fish or cheese for lunch?' suddenly seems an impossible thing to decide. Shopping is a trial in itself.

You could find your eating pattern disturbed as your appetite decreases because of the worry you feel. You may sleep less and take less exercise than before. If you smoke, that is probably the only thing which does seem to be on the increase, besides drinking.

But remarkably, despite the panic attacks and this general feeling of unease, you are probably managing to cope with your life. You may not be feeling particularly joyful about things, but you are coping. Overall, it appears that people who panic do manage to keep their social lives ticking over adequately, and don't allow the attacks to affect their working lives to any great extent – despite the incredible amount of stress which their bodies are having to cope with. It's amazing just how well most people do cope.

Avoidance

Because that first attack made such an overwhelming impact on you, it is small wonder that you are now so alert to the possibility of another. When, you don't know. But if you can avoid another one, you will. This is another way in which panic attacks can begin to affect your life. Nobody can blame you for not wanting to go into the supermarket, cinema or wherever you think you might come face to face with the panic attack monster (we could call it PAM for short!). It's like asking someone to walk willingly into the lion's cage at the zoo: not many people would want to do that by choice. It's not that you're frightened of the supermarket or cinema itself. You don't quake with fear because of the building. It's the thought of what might happen to you when you are inside which proves to be a bit tricky.

And so, in an attempt to avoid another attack, you 'learn' to avoid certain situations in which you have panicked before. This is why a large number of people who have attacks go on to develop agoraphobia to a greater or lesser degree. If you think this applies to you, you are not alone. There are an awful lot of people out there who share the same feelings and fears as yourself. Melanie remembers that 'I couldn't do or plan anything. It was controlling my life.' There is more about control in chapter 7.

So some people develop agoraphobia, some don't. You can have panic attacks without agoraphobia, but if you are agoraphobic you most probably have panic attacks. There isn't any way of telling beforehand who will develop agoraphobia and who won't, so presumably the possibility is there for everyone.

Agoraphobia is described in DSM-III-R (see page 12) as 'the fear of being in places or situations from which escape might be difficult (or embarrassing) or in which help might not be available in the event of a panic attack.' And so you may go into those situations you fear, but you couldn't exactly say you enjoy yourself while you're there. You will be feeling too anxious and worried about the possibility of another attack for you to relax enough to feel enjoyment. Jenny understands this feeling. 'I was frightened of it ever happening to me outside my home. But what frightened me just as much was the thought of it happening when I was with total strangers.'

There are a multitude of different potential agoraphobic situations: being on your own, being in a crowd, queuing, sitting on a bus or going on a train. Almost any situation in which someone has experienced a panic attack can become one which they start avoiding. One 16-year-old called Jimmy who experienced panic attacks felt uncomfortable on his own at home, which was where he first experienced his attacks. As a result the prospect of another one 'made me stay out much later at night, so as to be sure that someone was home.'

Obviously this can have a dramatic effect on a person's life. In Jimmy's case he could run the risk of finding himself in dangerous situations through being out late at night, and possibly cause untold worry for his family. Some people, because of their avoidance of potential panic places, have become housebound for years. Activities become more restricted as another attack happens in yet another place, adding itself to that lengthening 'Where To Avoid' list. For Melanie the effect was so great that it even disrupted her career as a dancer. Being unable to travel to auditions, rehearsals and classes, she now feels that she really missed out as a result. Similarly, Brian feels his panic attacks 'caused me to be deficient in some areas, like social contact, confidence. I believe these areas have prevented me from achieving some of my goals.' Without the practice of being in situations, you lose the opportunity to learn how to handle them successfully. Your confidence starts to go as you anticipate what you would call another 'failure'. There is more about confidence in chapter 9. It is important for you to gain control over your panic attacks before they take even more of a stranglehold on your life.

Besides learning to avoid certain places and social occasions, you may find yourself becoming uneasy during certain conversations. If you analyse them you will probably find they are those which bring on feelings of stress or excitement. So for example, you might find that hearing about earthquakes or wars are 'too much' for you. They make you feel jittery. Talk about illnesses or suffering makes you feel uneasy. Reports of surprises or exciting happenings can make you feel the same.

Anybody who hears these things makes a response: they frown and say 'Oh, how awful,' or beam a smile and exclaim 'That's absolutely fantastic!' You're just like everyone else and you respond too; but remember that your fight or flight response is primed, all ready to say 'Go' to another adrenalin release, and is looking for just the slightest provocation. Hearing any of those news items presses the firing trigger a little bit more. In feeling excited by the news your autonomic system discharges some more adrenalin into your system, and so off you go with the feeling of having another attack. So in your sensitized state, you may find yourself avoiding certain conversations or television programmes. It's all down to that adrenalin again.

Its Effect On You

As you feel more and more frightened, anxious, on edge and bewildered by what is happening to you, it is hardly surprising to find that not only has your ability to enjoy life decreased, but your self-confidence has taken a battering as well. You may have become demoralized as you felt the need to place more restrictions on your activities. Your friends and relatives may have become angry with what they see as you being negative or stubborn. (See chapter 15.)

Because of all this, a number of people who panic become quite depressed. Under the circumstances this is understandable, like Colin who said: 'They [the panic attacks) have made me tired and depressed and I have lost a lot of confidence as a result of them.' If each day becomes an endurance test – which you see yourself as failing with each attack – instead of a joy, it is bound to make you feel depressed. I would say this is quite normal. If it applies to you, take comfort from the fact that many others, like Colin, experience the same things as you. And I'm quite sure that anyone who went through these experiences would react in the same way. Just try to remember that experiencing panic attacks does come to an end. Re-read chapter 1 if you need more reassurance about that.

Worry About Potential Dangers

You may have read or heard bits here and there about panic attacks and worried that they have been linked to suicides. Let me put your mind at rest. According to the *American Psychiatric Press Textbook of Psychiatry* (American Psychiatric Press, 1988) the reported suicides may in fact be linked to alcoholism instead, because alcohol is used by some people in a misguided attempt to self-treat their panic attacks. There is no evidence to suggest that suicide is linked to simple panic attacks. However, if you have had suicidal thoughts, do go and see your doctor and explain how you have been feeling. The Samaritans (UK) or Befrienders (international) can also be an immense help at times like this. Ring them. Their number is in your local telephone directory.

You may be under the impression that panic attacks can induce fatal heart attacks. You may be worrying that your attacks are leading you in that direction. Let me reiterate what I said in chapter 1. No one has ever come to any harm or died as the result of a panic attack, and neither will you. The misunderstanding about links with heart attacks may have come about because of research which showed that a high number of people with panic disorder also have mitral valve prolapse. Although that may sound like a fatal condition, it isn't: it refers to a valve in the heart which, in simple terms, occasionally flaps the wrong way. It isn't fatal in itself. Rather, it is suggested that those who had mitral valve prolapse and died may have done so through 'normal' causes such as leading unhealthy, sedentary lives or through alcoholism. In general, people with panic disorder have normal health, so you have nothing to worry about. (However, if you have a real concern about your health, do go and check it out with your GP. That's what they're there for.)

The Effect of Panic Attacks on Your Health

Some people, for various reasons, have decided not to seek help and treatment for their panic attacks. What could happen as a result of this procrastination is that they develop other illnesses which are more 'visible' and which they do take along to their doctor for treatment. Of course, what happens afterwards is that other problems can emerge in place of the one which has been treated, or the same problem simply reappears later on. Because the doctor isn't treating the cause of the problem, i.e. panic attacks (simply because he or she hasn't been told about them), the real cure cannot take place. The sooner you openly acknowledge your panic attacks and start to take action, the better.

The Dangers of Self-Medication

In an attempt to treat panic attacks by themselves, some people resort to the use of alcohol or those illegal drugs which have a calming effect. Instead of seeking appropriate help, they resort to the bottle. Research confirms there is this link between panic disorder and problems with alcohol. We will look at this in more detail in chapter 10, but it is obvious that any relief it brings is only temporary and can lead to more problems than it appears to solve. Abuse of alcohol and drugs can not only affect your health, but if left unchecked can cause problems with relationships at home and work, can put your livelihood at risk and even your life. Self-medication in this way can have a devastating effect on your life. It isn't the way forward.

The Positive Effect on Your Life

Positive? Yes.

Because of an eventual recognition that all is not well, and perhaps out of a sense of frustration with what is happening to you and the way in which your life has changed for the worse, you may begin to reassess it. In my case, as I mentioned before, I recognized that although I was not sure what was happening to me, it was the result of something important. Through panic attacks, my unconscious self was trying to get the message across to me that all was not well. It appeared to be far more in tune with things than my waking, conscious self was – thank goodness! Eventually I listened and took the opportunity to re-evaluate my life. As a result I began to acknowledge that things were indeed amiss, without my having realized it. So I started to make changes. The same happened to Karen:

'Now I feel a lot stronger. I had to examine my life so closely to find out the cause of problems. I discovered things about myself I didn't like, so I began changing myself. Now things are better I'm glad I had to go through them.' That's right – she was glad she went through the experience of having panic attacks.

Theresa also says 'They [the panic attacks] have changed the way I acted and looked on a lot of things in life – for the better, I feel.' You may well be thinking, as you read it, that this is extraordinary. And I suppose it is.

Although panic attacks are extremely unpleasant, as are the associated feelings in between each one, remember that as well as attempting to protect you (through the fight or flight response), they are giving you the opportunity to find out just what is unsatisfactory in your life. I may be wrong, but I imagine that a person who is totally fulfilled in life, through their work and in their relationships, with no burdensome financial or other problems, is highly unlikely to experience panic attacks. When I reassessed my life, I realized that if I were somebody who was calm, relaxed, content and with few worries, I would probably not be having panic attacks. I gradually accepted that I didn't like certain aspects of my life which were causing me difficulties. Then I decided that I didn't want the attacks any more. But without having experienced them, I now wonder just how long it would have taken me to make that honest reassessment, and how much more I would have suffered in other ways as a result.

I see my panic attacks in a very positive light and, like Karen, I am glad I had to go through them.

And so panic attacks can indeed have quite a dramatic effect on your life in one of two ways. They can shut you in tight, into an ever-shrinking world in an attempt to hide away from them, or they can be seen as a way of giving you the opportunity to realize something important about yourself and your life. Attacks are an unpleasant experience for everyone, but it is up to you to decide how you will respond to them.

Summary

◆ Your sense of bewilderment, anxiety and unease is simply the result of becoming sensitized. It doesn't mean you are losing your grip or going crazy.

◆ In the face of the constant underlying stress and worry which you are experiencing because of the attacks, you are doing extremely well.

◆ It is understandable if you feel depressed or lacking in confidence. You're not alone. This happens to a lot of people who panic, and the issues are addressed in chapter 9.

◆ Be reassured: no one has died from a heart attack or anything else because of a panic attack.

◆ Alcohol and drug use and abuse is not the answer.

◆ Panic attacks can have a positive or negative effect on your life; it's up to you to choose which.

4

Why Me?

I hope that you now understand a little better what a panic attack is, and that you are reassured by the knowledge that attacks are a protective measure which your body is taking, and that although they are extremely unpleasant, you will come to no harm.

Knowing this is a relief, but it does not answer the question of why they started in the first place. You have probably asked yourself 'Why me?' at one stage or another. You may have asked your doctor why one person should have them and not another; you may well have received an unsatisfactory answer. To be fair, the reason is probably because there has, as yet, been no single cause identified which explains why panic attacks begin. However, there is a lot of research suggesting many possibilities. This chapter gives an outline of those findings.

In very general terms, researchers appear to fall into one of two camps. There are those who believe that panic attacks begin because of psychological reasons, and then there are those who believe that there is a biological cause for their onset. Below is a review of the recent discoveries in both fields.

Psychological

Perhaps the interest in panic attacks from the psychological angle developed from Freud and the psychoanalysts' interest in 'neurasthenia'. Although having a different name, this was probably the same as panic disorder. Modern-day researchers continue to look into the underlying causes and treatments from the psychological point of view, and through various therapeutic treatments, results have been obtained without medication. Since people have responded to this sort of treatment, psychological factors must have at least some bearing on why attacks begin in the first place.

Here are some of the factors which have been considered.

Personality

It is conceivable that there could be a panic attack personality 'type'. If there were, it could explain why some people have them and not others. Researchers in Italy studying anxious personalities appear to confirm this. They suggest that those people's feelings of anxiety could lead to the eventual development of panic attacks at some later stage.

Others have observed that people who already experience panic attacks tend to have certain shared characteristics. Being over-critical and disapproving of themselves is common, as is a tendency to have too high expectations of themselves. There are lots of 'shoulds' and 'musts' in their life, spurring them to drive themselves on and on. This stems from early childhood, when you learned to believe from over-strict parents that if you didn't do all the 'shoulds' and 'musts' you would have that all-important love taken away from you. This is a terrifying thought to children. Although this is obviously an inappropriate way to think as an adult, the lesson was probably learned so well that you are now quite unaware of it and the effect it is continuing to have on your life, as you continually strive to conform and to serve the 'shoulds' and 'musts' in your life.

Attributing successes to other people, while highlighting only their own part in failures, also apparently tends to be a characteristic of people who panic, as is blaming themselves when things go wrong. However, although introspective, they will also too easily immerse themselves in others' problems and readily respond to their needs and wants. In comparison, expressing their own needs is difficult. So they become worried and concerned about someone else's problems, and pile those concerns on top of their own which they try to ignore or deny.

Think about whether any of these things hold true for you. They are important factors to be aware of, since they are the sorts of things which can generate a lot of internal stress and worry which may weaken your ability to cope with other day-to-day problems. We'll have a look at this more in chapter 10.

Childhood Fears

Children are vulnerable and sensitive beings. Unfortunately, parents can tend to forget that, and unwittingly do harm by speaking and acting carelessly towards them. Psychodynamic theories suggest that if frightening situations make a great enough impact on children, unpleasant feelings and thoughts can be triggered later in adult life when they find themselves in a situation which reminds them of the original, fearful scene. It needn't be something which happened in real life; it could even be part of a fantasy. Disapproval, physical threats, and overwhelming stimulation could all be perceived by children as potentially dangerous situations.

Another incredibly frightening situation for a child to be in is where s/he fears separation from their mother figure. Initially this separation anxiety can show itself as school phobia. In later years the anxious feelings can be rekindled when the person finds themselves in a situation which reminds them, perhaps subconsciously, of that same threat. Panic attacks sometimes begin to occur after an actual or threatened loss of an important person or support system. Perhaps it echoes those early unresolved fears, but although these links have been suggested, it is unclear whether panic attacks are always linked to early separation anxiety or not. With or without the links with childhood separation anxiety, losing important relationships or other kinds of support does appear to predispose some people to panic attacks.

So it seems that incidents in childhood, the way we were brought up and taught to think about ourselves could all have a bearing on whether someone eventually in later life develops panic attacks. Subconscious worries and fears can establish, from very early on, a level of anxiety much higher than that of happy-go-lucky people. And perhaps because these anxious feelings have 'always' been there, this sort of person is quite unaware of them.

Life Changes and Life Events

Lots of research has now been done in the field of stress and stress management. It appears that it is not only unpleasant events in your life, like losing your job or a bereavement, which can cause stress, but so too can pleasant things. Getting married, starting a new job and taking a holiday are all potential stressors, even though they can be said to be positive and pleasant.

Bearing this in mind, some people experience their first panic attacks after important things have happened to them. Researchers have already identified the loss of support as something which can provoke the onset of panic attacks. Moving house, going heavily into debt, divorce, and any other major upheaval in your life may also have been responsible, especially on top of a generally higher level of anxiety which you may already have and of which you may be unaware. At the time when I started to have my first attacks I too was unaware of just how much stress I was under. Instead, I plodded along, taking things 'in my stride', then *wham*! Although I couldn't sense that I had reached my limit, my body's defence system did. Buying my first flat, changing jobs (into one where I wasn't particularly happy), my mother dying, and splitting up with my boyfriend are just some of the things which were happening all at the same time. I've since come to understand how much general anxiety I also have, so layering all those major problems on top, it is hardly surprising that my body decided that, with the stress and strain it was feeling, it had had enough. It alerted me to this through panic attacks.

Problem Solving Ability

Perhaps it is truer to say that life events and major changes are not in themselves the things which provoke the onset of panic attacks: how you react to them is much nearer the mark. Without good problem-solving skills, tackling life's ups and downs is that much harder, and this in turn will create more stress, worry and anxiety: a potent mixture for encouraging panic attacks. Constantly worrying about a problem without being able to reach a solution is a good way to keep anxiety levels high. Worrying is good only if it leads to resolution by taking positive action, asking for help, or by willingly accepting the situation as it is. If you don't ever reach that point, you run the risk of raising and maintaining levels of anxiety which could eventually overload the system, especially on top of high levels of background anxiety. Looking back, with better problem-solving skills I might have been able to divert the onset of my panic attacks by taking more positive action rather than simply coping with much that was unsatisfactory. And for me, 'coping' largely meant 'ignoring' or 'avoiding'. Consequently I lost my sense of perspective and could have benefitted from taking some advice from a counsellor, who would have been much more objective. I could also have developed some possible solutions to elements in my working life with which I wasn't happy.

Background Anxiety

People who experience panic attacks tend to have higher than normal levels of anxiety even when they are resting. As we have seen, it may be due to things which happened in their childhood, or it may be the result of too many long-term problems, or a combination of both. Chapter 2 explained what a panic attack actually is – the result of the fight or flight response springing into action. Feelings of anxiety, regardless of where they come from, begin to prime the body to make the same response again. The finger's on the trigger, ready to pull it at the least provocation. The whole nervous system has become aroused and is now highly sensitive. Thresholds for coping with excitement are much lowered, so even in a pleasant situation, if it encourages more stimulation, more adrenalin to be released, it is easy for the system to overload into a panic attack. Alternatively, relaxing can have the effect of releasing the block from feeling and responding to the heightened state of arousal, so suddenly, there you are in the midst of an attack. It all makes sense, really, doesn't it?

Misinterpretation of Bodily Sensations

Because of being in this highly aroused state, researchers also suggest that you become more sensitive to bodily sensations as you unconsciously look for the signal to actually start fighting or fleeing. Linked with this can be a catastrophic misinterpretation of what you sense. For example, you begin to notice your breathing, think it is too fast, unconsciously assume it's because you must be getting ready to cope with danger, and your body presses the panic trigger. Off you go again, trying to protect yourself from some imagined danger, this time simply because you thought the worst about what a harmless sensation could mean. We'll have a look in chapter 6 at therapy which has had some very good results in correcting this over-sensitivity and misinterpretation of bodily sensations.

Biological Causes

Lots of research into possible biological causes of panic attacks and panic disorder has revealed some interesting clues. However, no single cause has been identified, and the ones which have been of interest could be the result of anxiety, not the cause of it. For example, people with panic disorder tend to be more sensitive to pain, become more easily tired after exertion, and blood levels of lactic acid (which is a by-product from having exercised) rise to higher levels than normal. Although all of these could happen of their own accord, as it were, they could also be the result of stress and anxiety. Lactic acid, for example, is produced by muscles when a person is feeling stressed, as well as through exercising. So it all seems rather confusing in a chicken-and-egg sort of way.

Some researchers suggest that because panic attacks respond to medication, the underlying cause must be biological. Isn't this like saying that because cocaine can make you feel good, feeling good must always be caused by something biological? But let's have a look anyway at what some of their findings have been.

Heredity

Panic disorder tends to run in families. I was surprised to find out only relatively recently that one of my sisters experienced panic attacks a few years ago when she was undergoing a difficult time in her life. I also remember my other sister having what she can only describe as a 'funny turn' one evening at the cinema many years ago.

Because of this family link, researchers are now looking into whether it is a genetically-transmitted weakness. Recent studies have identified that there may be such a link, but they agree that their findings are only suggestive and by no means conclusive.

Until there is more indisputable evidence, it is just as feasible that the prevalence of panic attacks within families is due to upbringing and learned behaviour. And even if it does prove to be genetic, Elmer and Alyce Green, in their book *Beyond Biofeedback*, rightly say that although we may be genetically programmed at birth, it is how we choose to adapt and modify that programming which is important.

Organic Brain Dysfunction (OBD)

Figures vary widely for how many people who experience panic attacks or who are agoraphobic have OBD. Researchers in Edinburgh believe it may apply to a third of agoraphobics, but figures from USA quote 67 per cent – an incredibly high figure. So what is this organic brain dysfunction?

Babies are born with a number of primitive reflexes. As they mature, the reflexes become modified. However, some people maintain these responses which should have disappeared early on. An inability to bal-ance very well is a feature of OBD, as is cross-laterality. This means that instead of being, say, right-handed (i.e. predominantly leading with the right hand) and right-footed (i.e. predominantly using the right foot), a person with cross-laterality may be right-handed but left-footed or left-eyed and rightfooted. This can manifest as poor physical co-ordination. Visual difficulties are a feature of OBD as well; not whether you are shortsighted, but having poor eye muscle co-ordination or an inability to ignore movement on the edge of the visual field.

The effect of having these difficulties is to place additional strain on the central nervous system, making someone very vulnerable to stress. This could conceivably link in with the theory about misinterpretation of bodily sensations. Someone who unconsciously experiences some of these OBD-generated difficulties could, for example, feel wobbly on their legs, feel frightened, and start to panic – all in a split second. Not understanding what has been the cause of the wobbly feeling could be enough for someone then to feel fright-ened of it happening again, causing more anxiety and leading to it becoming a psychological problem too.

Since some of the symptoms of OBD are inherited, it could explain why other researchers suggest that vulnerability to panic attacks is genetically transmitted.

Interest in OBD appears to be growing, especially in its relation to both panic attacks and agoraphobia. It is possible to remedy the problem, and this will be discussed further in chapter 6.

Mitral Valve Prolapse

During the 1980s a lot of interest was stirred up because it was found that there was a high incidence of mitral valve prolapse among peo-ple with panic disorder. The mitral valve is a heart valve which should close once blood has been pumped through. In mitral valve prolapse the valve is sucked back on itself, like an umbrella being blown inside out. Through the stethoscope it is heard as a click-murmur and although it may sound as though it should be problematic, it isn't.

Despite the amount of research, no one has been able to explain the link between this and panic attacks. Whether high levels of anxiety cause the prolapse, or whether the prolapse causes panic attacks through misinterpretation of the heart murmur is not yet understood. The important thing for you to realize is that mitral valve prolapse, it has been discovered, is as common in the rest of the population as it is among people who experience panic attacks and it is a benign condition – it can't do you any harm.

Central Nervous System

As already mentioned, the onset of panic attacks tends to occur between the ages of fifteen and forty, with the majority beginning when people are in their twenties. It has been suggested therefore that they may be the result of an abnormality in the central nervous system, due to the fact that the noradrenergic system, which produces the hormone noradrenaline, may not become fully matured until adolescence and probably begins to decline in efficiency with age.

This possible biochemical abnormality could be the cause of panic attacks, but again research is, as yet, not fully conclusive. What they perceive as an 'abnormality' could possibly be normal if the person has high levels of anxiety, due either to difficulties they may have had in the past and which have not been resolved, or those they may be experiencing now.

Locus Ceruleus Theory

The locus ceruleus is an area in the brain which plays an important part in sending preparation messages to other parts of the body during the fight or flight response. The theory suggests that the locus ceruleus may be overactive in people with panic disorder.

It may be that there is a biological reason for it being so trigger-happy, or it could be that it is being overstimulated by other biological systems. If a person is highly aroused because of stresses and strains, couldn't this also cause the locus ceruleus to step up its activity?

Again, results from research are, as yet, inconclusive about this theory.

Carbon Dioxide Sensitivity

Martin Landau-North, in *For People Who Panic* (Anthos Park, 1985) noticed that the people he saw tended to be relatively inactive for months and possibly years at a time; especially agoraphobics, who may be particularly housebound. He suggests that this inactivity has the effect of lowering the carbon dioxide threshold. A certain amount of carbon dioxide is needed in the body for proper functioning. If it drops below a certain level, the body reacts in a way similar to a panic attack.

Klein, in his research in the USA into hyperventilation (see below) put patients in a room with 5 per cent carbon dioxide in an attempt to stop carbon dioxide levels falling while they hyperventilated. He found by accident that it had the effect instead of causing a panic attack. Following on from this observation, he then discovered that if he gave patients just two inhalations of 35 per cent carbon dioxide it was enough to induce an attack.

From this he suggested that people who have panic attacks are sensitive to carbon dioxide, perhaps because of an oversensitive smothering alarm – i.e. if you are being smothered you breathe back in the carbon dioxide you have just breathed out. If there is too much carbon dioxide in the air, Klein's suggestion is that you therefore think you are being smothered – and so you panic at this perceived threat.

I wonder if this could be one reason why people can have a panic attack in crowded rooms, or in places where there is inadequate ventilation? It also makes you think about the reported decline in air quality, especially in urban environments.

Hyperventilation

Hyperventilation means over-breathing. How can you breathe too much? When we are stressed, anxious, ready to fight or take flight, one of the things the body does is to breathe more rapidly, eliminating more carbon dioxide than normal in order to meet the anticipated demand for more oxygen for muscles to use. As already stated, we need a certain amount of carbon dioxide in our bodies and if it drops below that level it can bring on panic symptoms. Hyperventilating can therefore bring on panic symptoms through lowering the carbon dioxide in the body too much.

Hyperventilating may be not only a result of feeling too anxious; it can also be a learned breathing pattern formed in childhood, perhaps the result of an illness like bronchitis.

Breathing 'properly' involves the diaphragm, the sheet of muscle that separates the chest from the abdomen. You know if you are breathing correctly in the resting position if your stomach is moving in and out and your chest remains still. If your chest moves up and down, then you are breathing incorrectly, taking in too much oxygen and breathing out too much carbon dioxide – and running the risk of bringing on panic symptoms. Without realizing it you may be over-breathing all the time, provoking an 'inexplicable' panic attack.

If you are hyperventilating all the time, taking even mild exercise (which further reduces your carbon dioxide levels) will have a disastrous effect. Some people who have panic attacks say that exercise can bring one on and be confused as to why it has happened.

Studies have shown that when people with panic disorder hyperventilated on purpose, only 25 per cent reported panic-like symptoms, and the symptoms were less intense than an actual panic attack. This has led to new conclusions being drawn about hyperventilation. Instead of it being the direct cause of panic attacks, it could be that people misinterpret the bodily sensations which over-breathing brings about, fear that it might be an attack, and consequently bring on a 'real' one.

So although it appears that hyperventilating and panic attacks are linked in some way, no one quite knows whether hyperventilating is directly responsible for bringing on an attack, or whether misinterpretation of what you feel when you hyperventilate brings one on. Cowley and Roy-Burne in 1987 ended their research by concluding that perhaps both hyperventilating and panic disorder are part of an over-sensitive alarm system – perhaps because of too high a level of background anxiety, I wonder?

So while we wait for the researchers to decide, it might be worthwhile for you to start to take notice of how you breathe. We'll look at correct breathing patterns again in chapter 10.

Other Possible Biological Causes

Sleep apnoea is where breathing becomes obstructed while the person is asleep. Research has shown that there may be a link between that and panic attacks which occur during the night. If this happens to you, sleep apnoea may be the trigger which your hyper-sensitive system responds to.

Many women report the onset of panic attacks after **giving birth**. Melanie reported the onset of panic attacks at different times in her life. Looking back, the pattern which formed was obviously linked with the birth of each of her three children. There appears to have been little research in this area, and it is unclear whether the high frequency of panic attacks in women after giving birth is linked to endocrinological changes, or whether it is because of the stresses, strains and pressures which a new mother feels. However, some good news for women: an American study in 1990 showed that panic attacks are not linked to the menstrual cycle. They must be about the only thing that isn't!

Seasonal Affective Disorder (SAD) is where depression occurs because of a lack of sufficient sunlight. A recent report in the *Lancet* cited the case of a woman whose panic attacks decreased in line with the 'sunlight' treatment she received for SAD. This led them to wonder if there was a seasonal link with panic attacks. Do you have more in winter than in summer?

Off on another tack, researchers in Finland appear to have found a link between **gut flora** (the bacteria that live in the intestine) and panic attacks. Abnormal colonization in the colon, they believe, could have a 'pivotal role' in panic attacks. Certainly diet can be important in helping your body cope with stress and we'll discuss this in the chapter on lifestyle.

Conclusion

So where does all this leave us? Although the medical profession is agreed on what the symptoms of a panic attack are, they are unable as yet to agree on what causes them to happen in the first place. I can only speak from my own experience to draw conclusions and for me, I can certainly identify with a lot of what various researchers have unearthed. I think high levels of background anxiety formed the basis for my predisposition, perhaps because of how I was brought up. When the attacks started I was under an amazing amount of stress, losing a number of important support systems. I may also have a bio-logically inherited alarm system which is highly sensitive – good for me, it'll help keep me out of any more trouble now that I understand what it's about.

As with a lot of things, once you know the reason 'why', a lot of that fear of the unknown starts to disappear. Hopefully, through reading this book a lot of your fears will also disappear too.

Summary

◆ Researchers think that either psychological or biological reasons are at the root cause of why some people have panic attacks and not others.
◆ Since they are undecided, you could do some research your-self – on you. Start to have a look at your life and if any of the things mentioned could apply to you.

5

One Thing Leads to Another

The Cycle of Panic Attacks

Now we understand not only about what panic attacks are and how they can affect your life if left unchecked, but also what some of the possible causes might be. To complete the picture we now need to understand why panic attacks should keep on repeating themselves. Why don't we have just the one attack, like my sister, whom I mentioned in the last chapter? Most people, following their first attack, continue to experience one attack after another; if we investigate the reasons for this, we can better understand what can be done to stop them.

Your First Panic Attack

If we think back to the explanation of what happens in a panic attack, you will remember that what happens is similar to the fight or flight response, except that with panic attacks the reaction is not provoked by being in a 'dangerous' situation, although certain situations can later become associated with panic attacks just because they have already taken place there in the past. Adrenalin, the main hormone to be released, is a powerful force, making your heart beat faster, your muscles twitch in readiness, your breathing becomes more laboured. Now you know it is your body's way of getting ready to protect you, it doesn't seem quite so scary. But when you had your first panic attack you probably didn't understand what on earth was happening to you. As a result, because the feelings were so powerful and so frightening, you probably started to fear even the thought of having another one. Let's admit it, they're pretty unpleasant if you don't know what's happening, and because that first one came so unexpectedly and hit you with such force, you probably weren't looking forward to experiencing another one again. No one would.

When something which happens has such a powerful effect it can, after just one occurrence, establish what is known as a conditioned response in you. For example, if a person has been in a serious train crash, the effect on them could have been so great that now, at the mere mention of the word 'train' they begin to shake with fear. After that first attack you had, something similar began to happen to you. Because you knew how awful you felt, you began to fear having another attack. You started to worry in anticipation of the next. This is called anticipatory anxiety – worrying about the next attack, when it might happen, where you might be, and so on.

Over-sensitization

The physical force of that first attack probably shocked you a lot, making you feel quite incapacitated. With me, it crossed my mind that I might have eaten something which had violently disagreed with me, so all the next day I was mentally checking how well I felt. Did I need to dash to the toilet again; would I feel well enough to make it through that meeting; did I feel as if I was going to faint?

After the second attack, the awareness I had of my body was incredibly heightened. It had happened again, without warning as it seemed to me, so I put myself on the alert for the slightest sign that I was going to have another. In doing so I thought I would at least be ready for it when it came, although what I would then do I wasn't quite sure. And so I became sensitized to my own bodily sensations. Was that my heart beating faster again; was I starting to feel hot and sweaty; was that a feeling of lightheadedness? Interestingly, it has been suggested that this hypersensitivity to what your body is feeling could be the result of denying emotional feelings; feelings which may be unpleasant to acknowledge personally or which you feel others would find unacceptable. The suggestion is that if you ignore your emotions, theoretically you have more time, energy and mental space to concentrate on what your body is feeling instead. It serves as a useful distraction from the emotions you'd rather not acknowledge.

Escalating Anxiety

So we now have quite a powerful combination. We probably have a higher level of background anxiety (which we may or may not be aware of), we have the worry about when, where and how we might have the next attack, and we also have the anxiety about reading our body's signals. As a result you may find yourself saying 'What if . . .?' a lot of the time. 'What if I have an attack in the middle of that meeting?' 'What if I feel funny at the bus stop?' 'What if I have a turn and embarrass my partner in front of everyone?' 'What if . . . What if . . . What if . . .?'

With all those thoughts and worries going around in your head, perhaps without you being fully aware of them, it is hardly surprising to find that you are less relaxed than you could be. Stop to pause for a second – now. Are your shoulders relaxed, or are they tensed and up by your ears somewhere? What's happening with your forehead? Is it smooth and calm, or furrowed and frowning? And how is your jaw? Clenched and taut or relaxed and free? If you feel anxious and concerned about all those 'What ifs', then your body will respond accordingly. If you sit and watch a comedy programme on television, your body responds and you start to laugh. If you sit down and worry, your body also responds, but this time by becoming taut and strained.

What happens when you worry is that those feelings of anxiety start to prime the body for the next fight or flight. As far as your body is concerned, any worry must mean possible danger. It doesn't know the difference between a worry about your bank balance and a worry about a charging bull. Regardless, it begins to get ready to protect you from it (whatever 'it' is), so off go those hormones. Adrenalin starts to be released into your bloodstream – not much, but enough to have the effect of making you feel even more anxious, more alert to possible danger. The finger's well and truly on that trigger.

And so in this aroused state you go about your business, only dimly aware that all isn't quite as well as it could be, but not being sure why. You feel uneasy. You check again to see if it's the start of another attack. No, you're OK this time.

Stimulating Situations

Then you get into a queue at the supermarket. Supermarkets are stressful places with all that bustling and jostling, all those bright lights and bold display signs. It's easy for your sensitized system to feel overloaded. It already has higher levels of adrenalin than normal, and one of adrenalin's effects is to heighten all your senses. The reason for this is so that you can spot the first sign of any real danger. For example, if you walked through a forest after being told there was a monster in there which might attack, you would be highly sensitive to the smallest movement, the slightest rustle of grass, the faintest touch, just in case.

Similarly, the stimulation you get from being in a supermarket starts to send the adrenalin levels up even more. Remember that stimulation can be pleasant as well as unpleasant. Supermarkets aren't in themselves unpleasant places, but they are highly visually stimulating – they have to be because they're aimed at encouraging you to look and buy, look and buy. So the excitement you feel at being there automatically releases more adrenalin which, added to the higher levels which you already have is enough to press the trigger – the panic button's been hit, and off you go. It needn't be the supermarket, it can be anywhere where you start to feel more stressed: at work, in church, listening to the news, at home. But at the least provocation the system goes into action.

Even a small release of adrenalin is enough to make your heart start beating a little faster. You're very sensitive about what your body's feeling; watching out the whole time in case you start to notice another attack coming on. So now you start to feel more than just a general unease at being there (wherever 'there' is). You can actually feel something more physical – your heart beating faster. Instead of realizing that your heart's beating faster because you have become excited, and perhaps also because you're rushing to get back in time to cook dinner/watch your favourite television programme/feed the cat, you misinterpret what you feel. Or, to take another example, you could be enjoying an evening out with friends. One of them tells a very funny story and you start to laugh. Laughing tends to make you hot, but when you notice this you automatically think 'Is this it? Another attack? Oh no.' It is when you begin to think something like 'Oh no. This is it. Another panic attack', that you yourself press the trigger. Because you have misinterpreted your bodily sensations, you actually tell yourself that it must be an attack; that it is an attack. The supermarket doesn't press the trigger, nor your friend's funny story. Your thought does it. You do it. You give yourself an attack. This is discussed further in chapter 8.

Adding on the Fear

After the attack has passed, you think back over it. You remember where you were and what you were doing. For you it may be that it happened while out running, or when you were round at Tracy's house. Wherever you were when it happened and whatever you were doing will now become associated with having an attack. Remember about conditioned responses? You have just received another one with this attack. You would have felt it as another nasty jolt, and because again you could not explain why it happened, you do two things. The first is to associate the place or situation with having an attack. The second is to become more fearful. Your previous attack may have been when you were on a train, now it has happened in the supermarket. 'Why?' you ask yourself. You don't understand and so you start to assume it could happen anywhere, and begin to feel even more frightened. You realize you might not be safe anywhere. To you the attacks had no rational explanation and it is so easy to be frightened by the unknown.

So now we have more anxiety about the next attack. By now you've convinced yourself that you will definitely have another one – but you don't know when or where. This additional anxiety-booster makes you even more likely to have another attack even when you find yourself only slightly stressed.

The Cycle of Panic Attacks

The continuing cycle of attacks can be shown by the diagram in Fig. 1.

Given this scenario it is easy to see why a panic attack will happen again, not only because of your higher anxiety levels but also because of the triggers, the situations which make you feel more anxious, and because of how you misinterpret or 'catastrophize' your bodily sensations; you automatically think the worst when you notice your heart rate has increased. You wrongly assume it must be the start of a panic attack. In thinking that, you prepare yourself for one and lead yourself into it.

Agents Provocateurs

We all have our own triggers; things which set us off. Some you may be aware of and some you may not. It might be useful to have a look at this list of possible 'agents provocateurs', some of which you might not have known about before:

◆ **Coffee** More than two cups of coffee a day can bring on attacks in some people. A number of studies have confirmed that people who experience panic attacks are more sensitive to the

First panic attack

Increased
fear of next attack

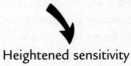

Panic attack

Heightened sensitivity

Thought cue: This must
be an attack

Increase in anxiety levels

Change in heart rate
etc.

Perception: I'm feeling
anxious so I must be
under threat in this
situation

Adrenalin release

Figure 1

anxiety-provoking effects of caffeine. It's certainly a powerful stimulant. Just two and a half cups of coffee can double the amount of adrenalin in your bloodstream! I've noticed this myself and now drink decaffeinated. Don't forget that tea also contains caffeine: about half as much as in coffee. So drinking eight cups of tea to replace your normal four cups of coffee won't really help matters much.

♦ **Alcohol** There is a high rate of panic disorder among alcoholics, and those who started to drink heavily before the age of twenty appear to be more at risk of developing panic disorder than others. As yet it appears unclear whether alcohol makes people panic or whether people drink because they feel panicky.

♦ **Drugs** Cocaine, marijuana, LSD etc. have all been linked to the precipitation of panic attacks. Jimmy identified smoking marijuana as being one of his agents provocateurs, as well as alcohol.

♦ **Smoking** Lots of people say they smoke to ease their nerves, but nicotine actually increases adrenalin production. The 'nerves' they say they have may in fact be due to the withdrawal effect of addiction to nicotine. Heavy smokers can increase their adrenalin by between 27 and 70 per cent. If you've been trying to give up, this may be good ammunition to help you stop. Certainly smoking would appear to exacerbate panic attacks, and at the very least it obviously isn't something which helps. You want to reduce the adrenalin in your blood, not increase it.

♦ **Medications for colds** A lot of them contain caffeine, which as you now know has a stimulating effect on adrenalin production.

♦ **Dieting or missing meals** Perhaps because the liver releases glucose from its store directly into the bloodstream if the body needs extra energy, missing meals could make you feel jittery. In turn you could misinterpret it as the start of another panic attack.

♦ **Having inadequate sleep** Not getting your full quota of quality sleep can make anyone feel jittery, and again perhaps these feelings are misinterpreted as the start of an attack. Missing sleep also puts an incredible strain on the body, and stresses of this nature can set off the release of those hormones again. Remember that your body can't tell the difference between being stressed from lack of sleep and being stressed because your chair's just set itself on fire.

◆ ***Exercising and relaxing*** We've already touched on these, but exercising could reduce the levels of carbon dioxide in your blood, even beyond the low levels they may already be at (due to hyperventilating, or stress). And as you now know, lowered levels can bring on panic-type symptoms. However, relaxing may also provoke attacks by removing barriers to feeling the effect of increased levels of adrenalin. Or perhaps relaxing gives you the opportunity to concentrate on your bodily sensations, which you are only too ready to misinterpret.

◆ ***Laughter*** Rapid breathing in and out of air may have the same effect as hyperventilating.

◆ ***Fluorescent lighting*** Adrenalin makes all our senses more acute, so fluorescent lighting could possibly be too much of a strain on the system, and be interpreted as a stress. And you know what happens when you're stressed. It would be interesting to see if people with OBD visual impairment (see page 36) find fluorescent lighting a particular difficulty.

Being aware of the possible effect of these agents helps. Nowadays, I'm careful of the amount of coffee and alcohol I drink. The last attack I had was so classic: a friend called round and we went out for a drink. I was tired and hadn't eaten but didn't feel hungry, especially when I became so excited about our topic of conversation. At the end of the very late evening I started to drink coffee. What a combination! Result: I think you can guess.

Here are what some other people have noticed about what brings on attacks for them:

'Thinking too much that another one may come on when I'm about to go out.'

'Being alone and quiet and hearing my heart beating loudly and then faster and faster. Also possibly caffeine, lager and marijuana.'

'Being on my own or going out on my own.'

'Stress.'

'Being given a complex task in a given time, for example exams. Answering questions in a group. Certain meetings with people – usually the first time.'

Some of these may sound familiar to you. In order to start to lick your panic attacks, you need to have as much knowledge as possible. You now have a lot of information about panic attacks, including why they repeat themselves over and again. Hopefully, all this will help reassure you and take away a great deal of that anticipatory anxiety. It is important to know why something happens. The other sort of knowledge you need to have is about yourself.

You are probably already aware of some of the situations which trigger attacks for you. Study the list of Agents Provocateurs and see whether any of those things could possibly be additional triggers. If there are other things, not on that list, which you suspect bring on an attack, include them in your own list. As I said, we all have our own triggers. For some it may be making love, for others it may be making cakes. We'll use this knowledge later in chapter 11.

Summary

- Without realizing it, you probably already have a high level of background anxiety.
- There are lots of situations which stimulate and excite us – either pleasantly or unpleasantly.
- Being stimulated releases adrenalin.
- Misinterpreting or catastrophizing what you feel makes things worse.
- Your own thoughts as much as anything can bring on an attack.
- You need knowledge. Find your own triggers; listen to your own mental cues.

Section 2

6

Solutions?

In chapter 4 we considered the different areas of current research into panic attacks. If you remember, it appears that researchers fall into one of either two camps: those who believe panic attacks have a psychological basis, and those who believe they have a biological one.

It is hardly surprising to find that the treatment you are most likely to receive will also tend to fall into one or other of these categories, and by far the most common is biological – treating the physical symptoms. The reason for this may be that when most people have their first panic attack they think there must be something wrong with their bodies – for example, a heart attack or a gastric problem – and so they instantly think of going to their doctor to check it out.

In this chapter we'll have a look at what tends to happen when people make that first visit to see their doctor.

The Consultation

You're worried and confused. You've experienced a funny turn, perhaps once or twice, and you can't understand what's happening. All you do know is that they terrified the life out of you and you feel jittery just thinking about what happened. Perhaps you haven't told anyone about them because one of the thoughts you might have had during the attack was 'I'm going mad'. And no one wants to admit to that, do they?

So you decided to make the appointment with the doctor, and there you are, feeling rather anxious because you're probably fearing the worst. As you sit in the waiting room, your worries start niggling at you with all those 'What ifs'. 'What if I need a heart transplant?' 'What if I am going mad?' 'What if it's some awful tropical disease?' (even though you've never been anywhere near the tropics).

Eventually the doctor is ready for you and the receptionist signals you through.

You sit down and start to explain in detail what happened: the shakes, the dizziness, the palpitations, the tightness in the chest, the sweating and the dash to the toilet.

The doctor listens carefully, perhaps looking through your notes and asking a few questions: had you eaten anything strange; how were you feeling beforehand, and so on.

Because a doctor is generally focused on physical complaints and causes, s/he will (quite rightly) think of any physical diseases and complaints which have similar symptoms and which could be the cause of the attack: thyroid problems, heart problems, low blood sugar or drug/alcohol problems, to name but a few. The stethoscope will come out, then your blood pressure will be taken. The doctor will ask you more and more questions in order to make the correct diagnosis. And as you field the detailed enquiries, it is natural for you to start to concentrate on what bodily sensations you felt at the time. Unconsciously, you begin to elevate these in importance in your own mind. You focus on them to the exclusion of everything else, and through the doctor's questioning you might even discover some 'new' symptoms as well.

The doctor is doing his or her job. S/he is trying to find out the medical (biological) cause of the physical symptoms you've just described in great detail. S/he isn't a psychiatrist or a psychotherapist, so it is to be expected that s/he focuses on your body in the way s/he does.

The Verdict

At this point, depending on your own doctor's knowledge, concern and abilities, they could decide to send you to a specialist for some more tests. They may not be fully aware of panic attacks or panic disorder and instead be more intent on finding out what could have caused the heart 'symptoms', gastric 'symptoms' or thyroid 'symptoms'. This lack of awareness could end up by causing you a lot of distress as more and more tests are carried out until, after trying in vain to isolate a physical cause, the doctor makes the correct diagnosis. This may have happened to you.

However, instead of sending you off to a specialist, s/he may well have realized that there is nothing physically wrong with you. You have a sound heart and everything's working as it should be. The verdict may come with some reassurance that everything is all right, but that you're probably a little run down/nervy/needing some rest. So now the prescription pad comes out, perhaps accompanied by 'I'll give you something to help you relax a bit.'

The Prescription

There are three different types of medication which have proved useful in blocking panic attacks. You may be prescribed any one of these. We'll have a look at each in turn, and the research which has been carried out into their effectiveness in helping panic attacks.

Tricyclic Antidepressants

Tricyclics have been around for over 20 years, being used mainly for depression. They have been well studied during this time and their side effects are well known to the medical profession: weight gain, transient jittery or 'speedy' feelings, constipation, reduction of mucus and sexual problems. Overdosage is dangerous.

Imipramine is the tricyclic which has recently received a lot of attention for use against panic attacks.

In terms of blocking panic attacks, imipramine is slow to take effect in comparison with the benzodiazepine alprazolam which is discussed below. However, although it is slow to take effect it does, over time, catch up and become just as effective. What tricyclics like imipramine cannot do, though, is to reduce those feelings of antici-patory anxiety about the next attack. So some people may initially be prescribed a benzodiazepine as well as imipramine.

Up to one third of people who take tricyclics will start to have panic attacks as soon as they stop taking them, and half the people who took imipramine in one study experienced significant problems with the drug. A staggering 84 per cent in total reported having expe-rienced some side effects.

Monoamine Oxidase Inhibitors (MAOIs)

MAOIs tend to be prescribed for people whose panic attacks don't improve with tricyclics. They are particularly effective with people who have phobias. Side effects are similar to tricyclics and, like them, they have a delayed effect. A quarter of people who take them also have the same jittery, 'speedy' feelings for 2 to 3 weeks. In addition, insomnia can be a problem and there are difficulties with them react-ing against some dairy foods, so you may have to make changes to your diet.

Benzodiazepines

Benzodiazepines have been used for around 20 years as a treatment for anxiety; Valium is one of the best known. Alprazolam is a benzo-diazepine which has recently received a lot of attention from researchers into panic attacks. Its biggest advantage over the other two types of treatment is that it is fast-acting. Improvements can be felt within the first week or two of treatment. It also reduces the anticipatory anxiety, which the other types of drugs can't do.

However, because the drug is metabolized quickly, it means that you have to take more than just one dose each day. It doesn't appear to have as many side effects as the others: feeling drowsy is the main one while it is being taken, although long-term use can lead to cognitive problems (ability to think) and benzodiazepines can be potentially dangerous for elderly people.

Researchers will quote many figures about alprazolam's effectiveness: 60 per cent of people panic-free at the end of an eight-week trial; 70 per cent with no panic attacks at all after more than two years of taking the drug. But effectiveness of treatment is now being looked at in terms of long-term use: half the people who use the drug need to be on it for at least six months; perhaps 40 per cent may need up to a year's treatment, and some 20–40 per cent could need to take the drug on a longer term basis. The relapse rate over the first two years is 20–30 per cent. However, informal reports of up to 80 per cent have also been quoted.

What they have also found out is that withdrawal and dependency can be a problem, as many who have been taking Valium or other tranquillizers are now finding out. And taking alprazolam for long periods can increase the risk either of dependence or of experiencing withdrawal symptoms when you stop. Gradually tapering off the dosage can help but even then, withdrawal symptoms may still be felt. It is also difficult to work out if what you feel when you stop taking them is a withdrawal symptom or a panic attack.

Doctors decide whether the side effects of drugs can be balanced against the benefits as they see them. It may be that someone is so debilitated by their panic attacks that they do need some respite from them, which medication could bring. However, I wonder if drug treatment needs to be the 'automatic', and seemingly only answer which some doctors can come up with, especially considering the side effects, possible long-term problems and the risk of relapse at some later stage. Figures appear unconvincing about whether any of these drugs are real cures. They may help people cope and they may bring relief, but for how long and at what cost? Recurrence of symptoms would surely indicate that drug treatment fails in truly getting to the root cause of attacks.

After the Consultation

You were perhaps told very little about what the attacks actually are. The doctor may not even identify them as panic attacks. You may have been given a few reassuring words that you don't have a heart complaint, but apart from the prescription now in your hand, you have been given little else.

What you ideally should have been given is information; a full explanation of what the attacks are. You should have been encouraged to understand what was happening to your body and your feelings. Instead of being guided towards helping yourself, you slipped into taking the patient, docile attitude which we are expected to take. The pronouncement was made and we were to play the game: take the prescription and report back, as expected, in a few weeks' time. That's that. Off you go and take one of these when it says you should do so on the bottle. The bottle ends up having more control over the situation than we do!

Another Possibility

Of course, it could be that you receive entirely different treatment when you visit your own doctor. You may find that s/he is able to recognize your symptoms straight away and make the correct diagnosis. Hopefully s/he will explain what panic attacks are and give you lots of reassurance that you will come to no harm because of them.

The doctor may still want to prescribe some medication for you. I would suggest, if this is the case, that you discuss it in great detail first. Make sure s/he goes through the pros and cons with you. Why does s/he think medication is necessary for you right now? What other ways are there to a) handle an attack, b) minimize the risk of having another one, and c) get to the root cause of them? Even if you are on medication already, you can still go back to your doctor and ask these very important questions.

Behaviour Therapy

In answer, s/he may suggest some form of therapy for you. If you have avoidant behaviour (that is, avoiding places or situations which you think bring on an attack) then s/he may recommend behaviour therapy.

Although medication can block panic attacks, it cannot 'cure' phobic avoidance, which many people develop. Behaviour therapy is commonly used to help overcome this difficulty. In a previous chapter I mentioned conditioned responses, when an experience is so terrible and frightening that it has the effect of making you avoid the situation again. This is what happens with a lot of people who panic. For example, they have an attack on a bus and because it was so unpleasant, they now avoid all journeys on buses and make other travel arrangements instead – or stay at home. Behaviour therapy aims to help you overcome these feelings of terror on entering situations which you think you prefer to avoid.

What happens is really quite straightforward. The therapist helps you talk about the specific fears and phobias you have. They help you imagine the situation and practise relaxation while you do so. The aim is to encourage you to go into those situations which you have been avoiding. You could be accompanied by the therapist when you do it, or you could be supported by your partner or a friend. Breaking through that fear barrier takes an awful lot of courage, and it may take a number of sessions with the therapist before you feel confident enough to take that step. Behaviour therapists say that without exposure to avoided situations, you will never find out how to unlearn those feelings of fright which surround them.

Behaviour therapy seems to work at helping to remove this avoidant behaviour. A report from Germany in the *Journal of Psychiatric Research* stated that reports on behaviour therapy, compiled over the last 20 years, show that it has been far more successful over long periods for the treatment of anxiety disorders (including panic attacks) than have drugs. However, it is far more common for behaviour therapy to be combined with medication. Some researchers suggest that this combination is the most successful form of treatment which has been studied. You can see its appeal. While the drugs are blocking the panic attacks, you can take advantage of the respite from them to build up your confidence in facing certain situations again. It teaches you how to cope. But coping and curing are two different things.

Coping is a way of learning how to manage a situation, learning how well you can duck and dive around the issues. It's like seeing PAM, the panic attack monster, still there but managing to hide behind the couch or wear a disguise to fool it, or only coming out when it's having a tea break. You may become very proficient at managing the situations, at coping, but PAM eventually comes back from its tea break and you have to carry on coping. Coping continues *ad infinitum*; curing ends things once and for all. Getting to the root cause of panic attacks is the only way to cure them. Researchers on the biological side are trying to find that root through designing new drugs to fit their hypotheses about what causes them. It appears to me that it must be like trying to find out what 'causes' a broken leg.

Psychodynamic Therapy

So you may be given medication or be sent to see a behaviour therapist, or both. The other option you may be given is to see a psychotherapist.

Psychodynamic therapy helps you look at the dynamic forces which lie within each of us: our wishes, feelings, conscious thoughts, unconscious thoughts and our fears. It posits that we feel anxiety because of some imagined danger which may or may not have originated when we were small children. This ties in with Klein's theory that people who have panic attacks do so because they may have experienced a great deal of fear at a threatened separation from their mother figure when they were very young. Losing supportive friends, family and networks in adult life can cause a great deal of stress and be one reason why panic attacks begin to happen in some people.

Psychodynamic therapy is often used by clinicians, but it has not been studied in the same way that medication and behaviour therapy have been. However, there are good reports of its effectiveness. For example, one report covered three case studies where treatment was solely based on therapy. No drugs were taken at all. Within 6 weeks of treatment, their panic attack symptoms had gone into remission; a result which is as good as those seen from taking antidepressants – and without the side effects. Therapy continued after the panic attacks had stopped, and follow-up – 2 years later in two studies and 5 years later for the other study – showed no relapse. They never had a return of their symptoms. They had no more panic attacks.

It appears to me that this sort of therapy gets to the root of matters. The other types of treatment may be valid in a limited way in helping you to cope, but you may still be left with a quality of life which is far from perfect (still wondering if PAM is going to come back from its extended tea break or not), and with too high a level of background anxiety. Psychodynamic therapy is one way of helping you see what PAM really looks like; where it came from; who or what it is. And in facing that monster you learn to see it for what it is – a squeaky little thing which you think has grown in size just as you have as you've grown older. But of course all that has happened is that your imagination has magnified it; the 'monster' is really just a tiny insignificance.

It's Your Choice

Any of these three options are yours. They are all available to you. You have a right to discuss each of them with your own doctor and s/he should be encouraging you to help you find the cure yourself, rather than expecting you to be the passive recipient of whatever written or verbal handout s/he chooses to give you.

Medication may be necessary; behaviour therapy may help if you have agoraphobic tendencies; but psychodynamic therapy may well help you get to the root cause and start addressing it.

More Options

OBD

I mentioned organic brain dysfunction (OBD) in chapter 4. At present it is not yet widely accepted as a cause although more interest is now being shown in the possibility that this may be at the biological root of panic attacks, in particular for some agoraphobics. Dr Weeks, consultant clinical neuropsychologist at the Royal Edinburgh Hospital, is currently researching into OBD and running a successful treatment programme aimed at correcting those balance and co-ordination anomalies which may lie at the root of agoraphobia.

Peter Blythe runs a private practice in north-west England which also focuses on OBD. His treatment is similarly concerned with correcting these dysfunctions through specialized exercises, tailored to suit your individual needs, which you can do at home. Regular check-ups are made until symptoms go into remission. Reported success rates are high: over 90 per cent in those who continue with the programme, according to Peter Blythe's own research and experience.

Cognitive Therapy

Unlike the other therapies already mentioned, cognitive therapy tackles head on the sometimes distressing thoughts we may have, especially about whether or not we are going to have another panic attack.

Cognitive therapy aims to change our misleading thought patterns which continually lead us into another attack because of their illogicality. For example, the therapist might ask: 'How do you know you are probably going to die when you have a panic attack?' You haven't died before, so how can you possibly know what dying feels like? A good point, you must agree. Cognitive therapy also helps you to reattribute physical symptoms to their correct cause; you learn to identify a racing pulse with enjoyable excitement rather than see it as a precursor to a panic attack.

Thoughts can be a great nuisance or a marvellous help. This is studied in more detail in chapter 8. Throughout the rest of the book you will discover the very exciting and important role you play yourself in becoming panic-free at last.

Summary

◆ Coping and curing are two different things. Decide whether you want to learn how to cope or how to cure.

◆ Accepting a prescription for medication to help you cope with your panic attacks is only one of the options open to you.

◆ You have a right to a full explanation from your doctor about what panic attacks are (although after reading this book, you may not need it).

◆ You have a right to discuss fully with your doctor treatment possibilities other than medication. It's your body and, equipped with as much information as possible, you can choose what sort of treatment it receives.

7

You've Got the Power

Power Play and Your Doctor

In the last chapter I brought up the issue of how we tend to fall into playing the docile, obedient role when we go to see our doctor. The majority of people do this. We tend not to be encouraged to take an active role in making ourselves better. Instead, we meet the doctor, answer his or her questions and wait for the pronouncement of either 'You're ill and this is what is the matter . . .', or 'There's nothing the matter with you; go away.' Then with little questioning on our part we accept the prescription or the dismissal, feeling that we must defer to what the GP says in all matters. So highly do we place them and their professional pronouncements.

In comparison with the doctor, we take a lowly, passive role. Even the word 'patient' has passive, non-active connotations, as though we should wait while others make us better. Indeed, that is what the system is geared towards.

Some doctors label inquisitive patients as 'difficult' and discourage them from taking an active part in their healing process. Who do you think would be labelled 'model patient'; the one who accepts without question, whether it be words, commands or pills, or the one who questions, challenges and tries to be more involved in what is happening to them?

Think about consultations. Who do you think has the power and control during them? I feel sure the majority of you will say that it is the doctor who is in control. Without thinking, we know what is expected of us from them (i.e. to sit quietly, answer obediently, accept willingly) and we play the game. Without question, we hand over the balance of power in the consultation about our health to someone else.

Effects of Feeling Powerless

It is interesting to find that a number of researchers have established a link between feelings of helplessness and depression. And we tend to experience as stressful those situations which we perceive as being beyond our ability to control. Because of this perception, our levels of anxiety are raised and the release of more adrenalin provoked.

Feeling that you have no real power over events has a very strong negative effect on you.

One of the most distressing aspects of panic attacks is their apparent unpredictability. When will it happen next? Where will I be? What if it happens next week at that party/tomorrow in the meeting/right now? Believing they come out of the blue in that way can make you very anxious – because you feel they are completely out of your control; that you have no power over them; that you are at their mercy. And so on top of the general anxiety you may have (but may not be aware of), and the worry about how awful the attacks feel, you also have the concern about when they might 'choose' to next catch you unawares.

People who experience panic attacks assume they are beyond their control.

Dependency and Independence

If you remember, one of the personality traits associated with panic attacks is dependency, perhaps originating from that hypothesized fear of separation from the mother figure. Anyone who is dependent will feel particularly vulnerable when they are stressed. They will want or expect someone else to take control, feeling inadequate to do so themselves. If it is true that people who panic tend to have feelings of dependency, then it would make sense why stressful situations lead more easily to panic attacks in them than in other people.

Witkin, in his studies of field-dependence – i.e. depending on things outside of yourself to too great an extent – also suggests that these feelings of inadequacy and lack of personal control can lead to many problems, including alcoholism. Interestingly, alcohol abuse has also been associated with those people who have panic attacks.

In order to gain control over our lives and what happens to us, we need to understand that we are separate from what goes on around us. We need to learn to be field-*in*dependent. External events happen within our environment, and we have little direct control over many of them. However, we do have absolute and total control over how we react to them. That is the important thing to remember. And once we have realized that we are separate from what is happening around us, we can then sit back and take a good, long, objective look at it all and start to see things in a better perspective.

Power Over Our Health

Just as we assume we have no control over the impact which external events have on us, we also assume we have no control over our bodies, and in particular our autonomous nervous system – the one which controls our panic attacks. We are taught that our bodies are in control of us; that we have no say in what happens to us in terms of whether we can stay healthy, or feel happier. We are encouraged to believe that things happen to our health in some mysterious way which has nothing to do with us. How can this be so? We are our bodies. And it is when our bodies become ill that we realize that we don't like having no power over them. But this is the price we have to pay for letting our bodies take over control. We have abdicated our real responsibilities. Left to their own devices, our bodies do as good a job as they can without being given any helpful guidance and direction from us. But remember that things in this universe have a natural inclination towards chaos and decay, unless you add another natural ingredient – free will; volition – and this comes from inside us. This is our personal power.

Controlling Your Body

Biofeedback is an excellent example of how we can learn to control our bodies. Electrodes are attached to various parts of the body according to whether heart rate, temperature or some other body signal is being monitored. Information which the electrodes pick up is registered by a meter, using light or sound, and provides a means whereby you can identify changes in your body as they happen. Watching or listening to the monitor feeds back information to you about those changes. You can come to recognize what the signals are like when you are either relaxed or excited. Through learning to recognize the changes, you also learn that you can will a change to happen without any stimulus from outside. So, for example, you can learn to reduce your blood pressure at will, or your heart rate if it is too high. Those things which you assume happen automatically are suddenly under your control. There are lots of astounding illustrations of what you can make your body do. For example, researchers at the Menninger Foundation studied a yogi who showed how relatively easy it was to create an external tumour, clearly visible beneath the skin, and then to make it disperse again with the same relative ease. That yogi is just a human being like you and me. There's nothing special about him or any of the people who have learned biofeedback techniques to control their bodies. The yogi is different only because he has realized and accepted that he does have ultimate control.

Pat Norris, who was researching into biofeedback for her Ph.D., also noticed that after a group had been taught how to control the temperature of their hand at will, they started to feel that they could perhaps control other things too, like emotions and feelings. Instead of being controlled by them, they began to see the truth: that they could bring an end to previously 'uncontrollable' behaviour patterns.

Your True Potential

It may sound quite extraordinary to you that we have this sort of potential; this amount of power. But if we bear in mind that we use only about one-tenth of our brain power, perhaps it begins to make a little more sense.

There isn't one person who realizes their fullest potential; genetic research now confirms this. So if the most intelligent among us are unable to achieve even a quarter of what they are fully capable of, it makes you start to understand what we could do if we did realize our potential power. We have the equipment, so to speak, but we haven't yet grasped (or perhaps been told) that we can do so much more with it. It seems that the way in which we use our potential at the moment is like someone using an incredibly powerful computer just to do simple addition sums.

Knowing that we have all this available to us is like suddenly finding that your bank account, which you thought was practically empty, (you were always too scared to ask what the balance was) in fact has a fortune beyond your wildest dreams in it! Just think what an impact finding that out would have. You would begin to realize that you could be and do whatever you wanted. Previous limitations would disappear. You would realize then that your destiny is far more exciting than you ever thought before.

Your potential is as big as that bank balance.

It seems a shame then that most people's remains largely untapped. Instead we use our energies to worry over day-to-day problems or in keeping internal conflicts alive. With panic attacks, the rational side of you is in conflict with what your body does when it has an attack. It just hasn't made sense to you why they have happened. Without understanding, your power to make any progress has been blocked. You have created that block through an inability (because of lack of information), or through an unwillingness, to realize your ability to do something about it. Too many people say 'I can't', too easily. Saying those words is instantly self-limiting and negative. It will get you nowhere fast. Reading this book will hopefully be the start of you saying 'I CAN' and distancing yourself from those negative others.

The Responsibility of Power

Beginning to realize that you have this potential introduces another element: responsibility. Through accepting it comes the potential for liberation. It means that you don't have to wait around passively for the Fates to determine things for you. Instead, you can make them happen in whichever way you choose, whatever is right for you. Ah, freedom at last.

But what a revolutionary concept this is! Society is geared towards us not accepting responsibility. Let's go back to the doctor's consulting room scenario. In that situation we are not encouraged to take responsibility for any illness. It is assumed that it has somehow happened to us, brought about by an outside agent, and that it is going to take another outside agent, i.e. the doctor/pill/therapist/surgeon, to make us well again. We appear to play no part in the treatment. We become, and stay, 'patient'. We abdicate our powers and yet again fail to seize the opportunity to realize more of our potential. Doctors don't encourage us even to try.

Your Power Over Panic Attacks

Besides acknowledging your potential I also think it's important to acknowledge fully that your body is yours. So are your feelings. So are your panic attacks. Who else's could they possibly be? And because the attacks are yours you can also choose to start bringing them to an end. You have the power to do so. Your potential for dealing with them successfully is truly enormous. The cure for panic attacks is within you, which is where all healing comes from. Just as our cells regenerate and heal an open wound, our 'nerves' can heal themselves too. You may decide to take help and guidance from outside, but it is still you who will heal yourself. No one else can do it for you.

This may be one of the problems with behaviour therapy. During treatment, the therapist instructs you to have a specific thought and then tells you how to react. They put you in a situation and then tell you how to cope. I wonder who has control; who feels a sense of responsibility in that situation? Ideally, therapy should guide and help you find your own way through by encouraging that important sense of personal power. Telling you to do something keeps you in that passive role.

All this is fine, you may be thinking. But how do I set about exercising this responsibility? How do I gain control of my panic attacks?

Exercising Your Power

Tapping into your potential and starting to exercise your power begins with accepting the fact that how you become from now on is your choice. You can choose to be free of panic attacks, or not. It is up to you. You may think you don't feel ready to take on the responsibility yet. That's fine. That is also your choice; but it too carries responsibilities.

In committing yourself to choosing that you want to be free of panic attacks, you then need to make sure you know them inside out. You may think you do, but how much have you remembered of chapter 2, which explained what happens during an attack? If you're not sure, re-read it now. Knowing the facts helps take away the fear. It helps you see PAM for what it really is, and to stare it straight in the eye and say 'I recognize you. You only came here because I've too much adrenalin in my blood.' It will already begin to cower at being found out. PAM is shy and doesn't like honesty looking it full in the face.

Then start to familiarize yourself with your own panic attacks. Have a good look at your recent ones. Think back to when they happened: where you were, what you were thinking, who you were with, what had happened just beforehand. Shutting out the memory of them is only suppression. That isn't the same as control, and nor will it lead to it. Instead, you need to hold them up to the light and see them from all angles. Become familiar with them instead of trying to shut them away. This may be difficult to do at first, but it is important. Be curious about them.

Acknowledge the feelings you experienced, too. Really get to know them. Try not to shy away from them. Remember it is you who holds the balance of power, not the feelings. They happen to your body, but your body is in thrall to you. Feelings can be difficult and you may want to turn away in your mind from them. To help you, remember that although you have feelings and that you experience things like deep anxiety, you are not your feelings. In the midst of my attacks there was always a 'me' who thought 'This feels awful. Am I going mad?' I may have been experiencing feelings which made me think of madness, but I was not that feeling. The voice which said 'This feels awful' was separate from the feelings, which had no voice at all.

When you fully acknowledge your panic attacks and really get to know all about them, you must then learn to accept them. By this I mean removing all your resistance towards them. In the past, you have feared them and tried to put up a barrier towards them (which you cowered behind). You tried to hide from the monster which you didn't know anything about but which frightened you. Once you know the nature of the beast you already begin to remove the fear. You know that no harm will come to you, so now if you have a panic attack you can accept it for what it is – too much adrenalin, and you can let it happen without resistance. Just go with it until it has worn itself out; until the hormone has finished swishing around your system. You know that trying to suppress it doesn't help, and only increases your anxiety. You know it will pass, so let it happen. Does it matter if you have a panic attack? It's unpleasant, but does it really matter now that you know it isn't life-threatening? At the moment you might probably think that it matters very much. In time, you will come to realize that it doesn't.

Acknowledging and accepting will take a while to happen. How much depends on you – we all go at our own pace. But since it takes three weeks to establish a habit and six weeks to break one (*Negaholics*, Cherie Carter-Scott [Century, New York, 1989]) you can see it may take time before the overwhelming fear of panic attacks stops. But time does pass and they will eventually be behind you. When I was at school and having to revise hard for exams (and hating it) I cheered myself up enormously by thinking that in two or three months' time they would all be behind me; even any disappointments about the results would be gone in time. Visualize yourself at some stage in the future, happy and without your panic attacks. Re-read chapter 1 if you would like some more encouragement that they do end.

Further Action

In discovering your commitment to change the way you are now, you give yourself freedom. Reading this book means that you are already making headway. Even before you picked the book off the shelf, you made the choice that you wanted to move forward and make progress. You were already looking for help; in this case a book. You were already starting to exercise your personal power.

You may decide that you would like to exercise it further by talking things through with your doctor again, this time on a different footing. Demand fuller reassurances from him/her if you still feel worried about anything you were told, or were not told. Be pro-active instead of simply reacting to what they say or do. Start to wield your own power by taking control of the discussion. It is easier to do this when you know exactly what you want to say, find out, ask about, and want, so prepare yourself beforehand; take in a written list with you if you think you might forget something. You have a right to have your questions answered.

If you still feel dissatisfied, you could always ask for a second opinion from another doctor, or ask to be referred to someone else who could help. Although you are starting to heal yourself, you might need or want additional support and guidance. Think of that help as a tool for you to use. You stay in control of it. Tools don't control you.

And in reading the rest of this book, hopefully you will start to develop an even greater awareness of how much more you can do to help stop your panic attacks once and for all, beginning with the next chapter which looks at the power of thought.

Summary

◆ Lack of control creates stress.
◆ You have a vast potential to control any aspect of your body, mind or emotions.
◆ Your body, your feelings, and your panic attacks belong to you.
◆ Your panic attacks are your responsibility and no one else's.
◆ Acknowledge and accept them.
◆ You have the power to change them.
◆ The choice of whether you exercise that power is yours.

8

A Thought is a Thing

In the last chapter we started to look at the potential power we all have within ourselves, but which we rarely fully use. We looked at the power of choice, and how you can start to exercise your control over your panic attacks. Now we will go one step further and discover how your potential power can be tapped even more.

A few years ago I was on holiday in Cornwall and came across a museum of witchcraft. Among the exhibits was a section on spells (of course). Accompanying displays explained the basis on which they worked, which was fundamentally that 'a thought is a thing'. It was their simple way of describing the power of the mind. They understood that thoughts can be powerful enough to bring about real changes in people's lives.

This concept is also to be found in a wide range of literature including business, religious and medical texts. It appears to underpin a lot of issues, including panic attacks.

Your Perception of Situations

Thoughts are powerful things. Of that there is no doubt. I can use myself and this book as a simple example. Before writing each chapter I am faced with a mountain of notes and references which I've collected. They are in no particular order. If I attempted to start writing from the jumbled notes straight away, the job would be immensely difficult and cause me a great deal of anguish and anxiety. However, if I organize the notes first, thinking carefully about which to use, which to discard and what should go where, the anxiety disappears. The thoughts organize the notes which then has the effect of making me much happier about putting pen to paper.

Alternatively, I could have treated the situation differently. I could have looked at the pages of photocopies and scribble and thought 'Heavens, I can't write anything using this,' and promptly walked out of the room not having achieved anything, or just sat down in despair, and become quite depressed about it.

The same situation can be perceived and thought about in different ways. The situation is not the thing which affects us, although we are brought up to believe in that idea. If it were so then all situations, all happenings, all events, would have the same impact on everybody – and they don't. For example, when taxes are increased one person may feel upset at how much they are going to lose out of their salary. Someone else, say a person with a disability, is happy because it means the money will now be available for government schemes which will assist them. We all have different sets of personal circumstances through which we interpret events in our own individual way.

Perhaps Hamlet summed it up the best in saying, 'There is nothing either good or bad, but thinking makes it so.' We can choose to have bad thoughts about something, or we can have good thoughts. Each will have a different impact on us, and the choice is ours which one we want. Someone who goes through life with positive, optimistic thoughts will generally have a happier time than someone else who does the opposite. One person leads a full, enriching life, open to new experiences because they think 'Yes,' to as many opportunities as they can. Someone else thinks 'I can't do that' to any chances which come their way. They limit themselves and become who they already think they are. You have the equally valid choice to remove those limits and become who you would ideally like to become instead. It only takes a thought.

Your Thoughts and Your Body

So what foundation in fact has all this? Hippocrates, a Greek physician some two thousand years ago, understood well that the body and mind are inseparable. How healthy your body is depends on your state of mind, and vice versa. For example, you now know that worry and anxiety release lots of damaging stress hormones. Conversely, meditation and mental relaxation can have a powerfully soothing effect on the body. Hippocrates knew this too, but science only now seems to be catching up with him.

Cyberbiology is the name of the science which studies self-regulation, i.e. how we can make our bodies do what we want through directed thought. Meditation is one well-known method. Cyberbiologists have been studying this as well as other techniques such as biofeedback, yoga and guided imagery. Because meditation affects metabolic activity, it has been suggested that it may be useful in learning to control anxiety. It has been found that it significantly decreases the levels of blood lactate, an excess of which makes you feel panicky. (Injecting a person with sodium lactate is one way of testing to see if the symptoms he or she reports are due to panic attacks. If they are, the person begins to panic after the injection. If the symptoms are due to some other cause, the person does not panic.)

One interesting experiment carried out by Oosterhuis in Amsterdam illustrates well this link between mind and body. He studied 500 people who were experiencing physical pain for which no explanation could be found. His astounding results showed that out of 331 who complained of pains in the neck, 329 of them also had feelings of aggression. Of those who had feelings of fear, nine out of ten of them had pains in the abdomen, and six out of ten of those with unexplained lower back pain had feelings of despair. Statistically, these figures speak volumes, showing a strong link between one's emotions and how they can detrimentally affect your body.

A similar finding was made in London's Westminster Hospital, where a study of people with rheumatoid arthritis revealed that the disease tended to begin soon after the patient had experienced a major upset in his or her life. The study also showed that an over-powering mother figure was also a common element in their back-grounds. Both of these have a strong emotional impact on a person. So it would seem to suggest that the emotional upheaval manifests itself as pain through rheumatoid arthritis.

We have all heard stories of people dying of 'a broken heart'. Matthew Manning, in his book *A Guide to Self Healing*, illustrates an example of this with the story of a woman whom he had been treating for cancer. She was responding well and making good progress. Then her daughter, to whom she was particularly attached, was killed in a car accident. Within six weeks the patient too had died. She thought she had nothing to live for.

Giving yourself cues or thoughts like this one has a powerful effect. The human body responds to whatever message we give it. It's as though our brains are like computers which we program. Like any computer, the brain does not decide whether it likes the message or not; it is capable only of accepting commands and acting on them. So by repeatedly saying, and believing, something negative like 'Everyone in my family goes grey by the time they're thirty,' programs the brain to make the body do the same. We must be careful how we program ourselves. It's like the wise warning 'Be careful what you ask for; you might get it.'

Positive Thoughts

However, that's looking at the effect of negative thoughts. Positive ones have similarly remarkable effects – and much more pleasant. I just mentioned grey hair. In Elmer and Alyce Green's *Beyond Biofeedback* there is an account of how one man made his grey hair return to its former brown colour just through thought control. He spent time every day imagining his hair the colour it used to be. And it worked. It did take seven years, but the important fact is that he made it happen – simply through the power of thought.

On a more serious level, Norman Cousins' experiment on curing himself of a potentially fatal illness is now well known, and documented in the book *Anatomy of an Illness*. Instead of accepting the passive patient's role, complete with full medication programme, he decided to treat himself. Part of this involved taking large doses of vitamin C; the other of watching comedy films. The laughter proved to be an essential ingredient in his recovery. Positively stimulating his mind was as important as feeding his body.

Drs Carl and Stephanie Simonton also use positive 'programming' in the management of another potentially fatal illness: cancer. They use creative visualization, developed as a result of studying reports of some 400 people who had experienced spontaneous remission. The one common element to explain this 'mysterious' happening was a change in attitude which always involved positive emotions, feelings and thoughts. The creative visualization the Simontons use encourages such thoughts and a positive frame of mind. Their results show that it works.

Studies indicate how this might happen. Scardino, a researcher, found that after relaxation and use of visualization, the number of natural killer (NK) cells increases. These cells are part of the body's immune defence system, and kill the potentially dangerous cancer and virus cells. So now there is a more scientific explanation to justify the Simontons' work. It also means that thoughts really do make things happen in a very real sense. In this case, it makes 'good' cells appear from nowhere – as if by magic. A thought is a thing: in this case, cells. It makes you think again about 'miracles', doesn't it?

There are other simple examples which show how thoughts affect your body, like bridge workers or builders on skyscrapers who do their work successfully because they don't think about the risk of falling. Without the thought they are unlikely to do it. But if they start to worry about it they increase their likelihood of an accident, as their anxiety levels rise and begin to make them feel dizzy or shaky.

There are also reports like the one about the seven stone woman who lifted a tractor because her son was trapped underneath it. In this case the thought and emotion were so strong that it was enough to galvanize her to do a 'super-human' feat. (*The Joy of Stress*, Dr Peter Hanson [Pan, 1987])

Placebos

I also want to mention placebos. These are sugar pills or other inert substances which are given to people instead of active drugs. They are most commonly used in drug trials; one group is given the 'real' pill and the other the placebo, to see whether the drug on trial is any more effective than a bogus one. Astoundingly, there are always some people who respond to the placebo. It has the same effect on some people as 'real' medication. So why isn't everyone taking placebos instead of drugs which have side effects?

Studies over the last twenty years have documented this placebo effect well. They are discovering that thinking and believing that something will work, often has the same effect as taking a drug which will do it for you. Placebos work, and do so because people think they will.

Your Thoughts and Your Panic Attacks

So what has all this to do with you and your panic attacks, you may be wondering? Well, it's important for you to realize the impact that your thoughts have on your body. They aren't separate things which happen only inside your head. Thoughts happen to the rest of your body too. This applies to panic attacks as well.

It's also important for you to realize that your thoughts don't come from somewhere over which we have no control. You make your thoughts. It is you who decides what to think.

Your first panic attack will have happened spontaneously, and probably be the result of over-excitement (physical or mental), or of too much anxiety and worry (conscious or unconscious). Negative thoughts would have played a part. Positive ones are unlikely to be involved in a panic attack. Also, as we have already seen, because the experience frightened you so much, you started to fear the next one. This is where your thoughts really began to have additional impact.

Because of this fear, each time you felt a little hot, you started to think 'Oh no, another attack!' When you next noticed your heart racing a little, you instantly thought 'Here we go again.' Because you were so on edge about another attack, and focused on it all the time, scanning your body for the least sign that another one might be happening, your thoughts became centred around having another attack. Anticipating another one (through thinking about it) is almost the same as having one. A thought is a thing.

Looking back at the diagram in chapter 5 of the cycle of panic attacks, perhaps you can understand the importance of the initial signal even more now. 'What if I have an attack?' is a powerful thought and starts to program your brain to expect another one. It's on the look-out – and ready. The anxiety level rises because of the thought, adrenalin levels start to increase, then your heart rate, and off you go again. If you hadn't had the thought 'What if . . .' in the first place, you would be unlikely to have had a panic attack at all.

But imagine you are in a situation where you have started to feel uncomfortable and as a result had that very thought, 'What if . . .' or something similar. If, for example, at that moment the only other person in the room shouted for help in extreme distress, your attention would be taken away from your potential panic attack and your thoughts would then become focused on the other person. Under such circumstances I think it would be unlikely that your panic attack would happen. It wouldn't be receiving any more cues to feed it into action. Initial thoughts generate only a potential panic attack; it isn't inevitable. Between the feeling of discomfort and your reaction (i.e. a panic attack) is a thought. This is the troublesome little piggy in the middle which decides whether you have a panic attack or not.

Using Your Thoughts to Help

Some of you may be confused by all this talk of thoughts which you have and which provoke attacks. A lot of people initially say that they don't have such thoughts. Aaron T Beck, who developed cognitive therapy, confirms that many people are unaware of these seemingly automatic thoughts. They do happen very quickly, and sometimes without words. They can be images or sensations, which are less specific than words. Nevertheless, he assures us that we all have them. The trick is in catching them. Unless you know what the thoughts are, it is difficult to do something about them.

So next time you begin to feel uncomfortable, focus on what is going on in your head and listen to what your own thoughts say. It may take a few attempts, because the thoughts are so quick and so instant in their effect that a panic attack can happen almost before you realize it, which is what makes you assume they are spontaneous. But with practice you will eventually begin to catch that butterfly thought.

Once you know what it is (you may have a selection which you use on different occasions), you can start to investigate. What happened just beforehand to make you think that particular thing? Why does that thought occur rather than another? Why do you assume it is true? Is it true?

It may be that your thought is about a bodily sensation, such as feeling faint, or breathing hard. This reminds you of your last panic attack and so your thought may be 'I feel rather faint, I must be having another attack,' or it may go straight into 'Here it goes again. Another attack.'

Another type of thought you might have is about dying, losing control, or going mad. These too are just thoughts, and are generated in response to the bodily symptoms you feel. Because you have found them so distressing and extreme you assume you must, in fact, be dying, about to lose complete control, or that you really must be losing your marbles to feel this awful without any reason.

All these thoughts are generated by you. You feel a certain way and so you play the same record again; the one which always plays before you have an attack. You are constantly reinforcing the message every time you notice the feeling. You can only stop the record, stop the thought, if you can first identify it. Then you can look at the thought and really question whether it is appropriate or not.

For example, feeling hot and breathing heavily leads you to think of a panic attack. Being in a stuffy room affects everyone in that way, but you misinterpret the feelings you have for a panic attack. Others in the same room, feeling the same, think 'Gosh, it's hot in this room. It's making me feel sweaty. You really can't breathe.' They may then suggest that someone opens a window.

Around at a friend's for coffee and cakes you begin to notice your heart beating very fast. Again you may misinterpret it and think 'Oh no! Not here! Not an attack right now,' and off you go. Someone sitting next to you also notices her own heart pounding in the same way but thinks 'I'm thrilled about seeing these people again. I haven't seen them for ages. There's so much news to catch up on. I'm really excited. Perhaps I'd better not have any more coffee because it makes me feel too jittery.'

This is the same situation, affecting two people in the same way, but they interpret their sensations completely differently; one positive, one negative.

Another example could be a business meeting. You feel uncomfortable because you're not sure about how you will perform. You've a difficult boss who hasn't given you much encouragement since you and your colleague were both promoted. Knowing you have to speak, and speak well, brings on a high level of anxiety because you feel the boss will be looking for fault. You start to have a panic attack when you notice you are sweating hard.

Your colleague is also having a hard time in her new position but realizes that the boss finds it difficult to give praise. To make sure she is doing OK, she made an appointment with her to talk about her progress and to find reassurance. However, she too is still anxious about the important meeting, but thinks 'This is going to be tough. I hope I perform well. Ms Boss says I'm doing all right, so I can only try to do my best. Gosh, it makes you hot under the collar, though.' These thoughts don't lead to a panic attack.

In all these situations, there are two ways in which you can turn your thoughts. You can interpret what you feel as a precursor to a panic, or you can reattribute it to the proper cause, e.g. you're hot because the room's too hot. There is also a negative and a positive way in which you can interpret the situation: as exciting or threatening. Remember that adrenalin is released with any stimulation: good or bad. It's up to you how you choose to interpret what you feel.

Cognitive Therapy

Cognitive therapists progress through this sort of analysis with their clients. Unlike psychotherapists, who tend to look at relationships, unresolved inner conflicts and emotional issues, cognitive therapists attempt to identify current thoughts which are adversely affecting someone's behaviour. You may decide to exercise your personal power and ask your doctor to refer you to a cognitive therapist. Use them as a tool for learning how to think in more appropriate ways to help stop your panic attacks.

Affirmations

A French doctor called Emile Coué successfully treated thousands of people with affirmations. Affirmations are positive statements, simple and clear, which are spoken aloud or thought silently to yourself. They are a way of reprogramming our brains with new thoughts. His famous affirmation is 'Every day, and in every way, I am getting better and better.' Rheumatism, paralysis, ulcers, and even some tumours were positively affected by this simple sentence being repeated by the people who came to see him.

A thought is a thing; it is also immediate. Once you notice the thought which you have prior to your panic attack, you will realize how fast-acting it is. This is an exciting realization. It means that positive thoughts must also be instant in the effect they have on you. You can start to be positive with just one thought, right now. You can start to make progress from here.

Use Coué's affirmation above, or have some fun making up your own. They need to be positive, in the present tense, simple and appropriate for you. Here are some examples:

◆ I am feeling good.
◆ I am calm and in control of my own thoughts.
◆ I have the power to make myself better.
◆ I love myself and my body.
◆ I feel strong and positive.
◆ I enjoy feeling excited.

You can use affirmations throughout the day to 'recharge your batteries' and to help you maintain a positive frame of mind.

Self-statements are similar and can be used to help avert an attack. For example, you could say 'I know my heart is beating fast, but it will eventually slow down again.' 'I feel jittery, but it is only because I have too much adrenalin in my bloodstream just now. It will eventually fade away.'

Now that you know why you feel the way you do, you can make your own self-statements for you to say to yourself. They will have the effect of reminding you about the real reason why it is happening, take away that feeling of fear, and help to calm you down. Eventually you will find that the sensations you experience begin to matter less and less as the re-programming starts to take effect. It may not happen immediately, but be assured that happen it will. And all because of a thought.

Summary

◆ There are lots of real examples to confirm that a thought really is a thing.

◆ You have complete control over your thoughts. They don't just happen or come from somewhere else.

◆ You have an immense amount of power to be who you want to be. And it all starts with a thought.

◆ Your thoughts cue you into an attack. Find out what those thoughts are, realize their inappropriateness, and find more appropriate ones.

◆ Affirmations help re-program your brain.

◆ If you would like some help with your thoughts, exercise your personal power to ask for a referral from your doctor to see a cognitive therapist; a tool for you to use to help yourself even more.

9

Confidence, What Confidence?

As you know only too well, panic attacks can have a devastating effect on your life. The constant threat of yet another one has you on edge the whole time, making matters worse because raised anxiety levels put you more at risk of actually having one. I hope the last chapter gave you lots to think about in terms of how much potential power you have in being able to avert those anticipatory, provocative thoughts. Remember that you don't have to try to control anything. You already are in control. It's your choice which thoughts you decide to have.

Your Confidence and Panic Attacks

Hopefully, realizing this will start to have a positive effect on you. But you may still be thinking a negative 'I can't do that. I can't even go to the cinema without having a wobbly.' Knowing that you can start to change negative thoughts such as that one helps, but in the meantime it is highly likely that your confidence is quite low and holding you back from the thought of trying. Panic attacks have this effect.

This is how some people responded when asked what their confidence was like during the time they were experiencing their panic attacks. Their answers were remarkably similar. Perhaps yours might be, too:

'None.'

'Almost none.'

'Hardly any at all.'

'Not a lot.'

'Not very much, I'd say.'

'Very little, if any – my husband used to tease and call me a "neggy": negative. Now I am getting there. I give things a chance before I say I can't do this or that.'

All these people's confidence was affected through having panic attacks. It's understandable why. If you are regularly struck by overwhelming physical and mental symptoms which you aren't able to understand or explain, it is bound to be a blow to your confidence. Normally, you know exactly how you are going to react in a situation. For example, going to the cinema: you have an ice-cream, perhaps; you sit and watch the film for two hours or so; you leave the cinema; you talk about the film; you go home, or for something to eat. That is what normally happens. Suddenly you find that what you confidently expected to happen doesn't. All at once you feel hot and panicky and you just have to leave the film half way through. Your partner is as confused as you. The evening's entertainment is cut short, leaving you with the thought that you really don't know what to expect next time. You think that you must have been wrong in your expectations, so your confidence in your ability to pre-judge a situation goes down a notch.

Similarly, your confidence in being able to 'handle' the same situation next time in any better way now comes into question. You feel that you can't take it for granted any more that when you go to the cinema it will be an enjoyable experience or that you will be able to see all of the film. Instead, you may disrupt the evening, and spoil your partner's enjoyment, too. And the more times a panic attack happens, without you being able to understand why, your confidence takes another beating until eventually, if things become so difficult, the only confidence you do feel is in predicting that a panic attack will happen.

Through a greater understanding of what panic attacks are all about, I hope you are now feeling a little more at ease about them. The fear of not knowing what they are is behind you. And as you become more sure about the facts, you can already start to feel more confident in knowing that you will come to no harm, that they will eventually go away, and that you have a great deal of power over them. You can begin to feel more at ease, and yes, confident about the next one. You have already made progress now in knowing these things.

But until they eventually stop, you can help yourself make even more progress by improving your undoubtedly flagging self-confidence in other ways.

Know Thyself

These were the words over the entrance to the oracle at Delphi; and what wise words they were. They are a reminder that in fully knowing yourself, you can discover that the answers are indeed within. This applies to self-confidence as much as anything else. In knowing yourself you can feel confident about yourself, and so find the answer within you. If you don't know anything about You, how can you ever feel confident about being with yourself? People are rarely fully confident with strangers, but with friends they are more at ease. So if you are a stranger to yourself, you too are likely to feel less at ease or confident than if you were friends with You.

So how much do you know about You? You may have lived with You for a long time, but how aware of your good and bad points are you? Perhaps because of upbringing, perhaps because of our society, we are inclined to concentrate too much on only our deficits.

Chapter 4 commented on the tendency in people who panic to have some shared characteristics. One of these was an inclination to be over-critical and disapproving of ourselves. For whatever reason, this may be true. Have an honest look at yourself and see whether it is or not. Doing this is difficult, because we are taught not to think too highly of ourselves – pride is a sin, etc. But we tend to weight the balance too far in the wrong direction. We look at ourselves and see only things to criticize. Criticism is fine if it is constructive; being critical about yourself without cause and reason is destructive and will only help to erode your confidence away. Instead, we need to look at ourselves, get to know ourselves so that we can a) appreciate the good things about us, b) start to change those things which we don't like, and c) learn to accept those things which we can't change.

Start off by having a look at your abilities. And I positively reject any claim of 'I don't have any.' If you can bake a cake, prune flowers, balance your bank account, or make a decent cup of coffee, then you already have abilities which I envy. I could concentrate on those particular deficits in myself, over-generalize, and say 'Because I can't do those things, I can't do anything,' but I know that would be untrue. I find it difficult to do some things very well, but I can certainly do others. In this spirit, start to have a long look at what you can do and what you find difficult. It's important to know both, because none of us is perfect. We can't be excellent at everything. But we do need to keep our sense of perspective about what we can do, about what we have achieved. We tend to keep our sights on the future and what we haven't yet done, forgetting to look back and appreciate how much we have already achieved which we can feel good about.

Make a list of your abilities. Turn your mind to different areas of your life: work, home, relationships (with children, elderly people, partners, friends, strangers, relatives), leisure activities. Try to bring your mind into sharper focus. For example, you may take your abilities at work for granted and focus only on what you find difficult, forgetting that you are excellent at organizing office parties and understand the intricacies of the photocopier like no other. Look at the things which you know you are good at. What do people compliment you on? What do they ask you to do because they know you will do it well? And what do you enjoy doing? If you enjoy doing something, then you tend to be good at it. It's all right to admit to enjoying doing something. It's also all right to admit being good at it.

Let your mind roam free. No one else need see your list. Indulge yourself and add as many things as possible. Still only one or two items under Can Do? Then look at the other list again. See if you can rewrite them in a more realistic way. For example, I could have put down 'I can't ride a bike.' A truer way for me to write it would be 'I can't ride a bike right now, because I've never tried. When I do try, I may find it difficult at first, but I can practise and may improve.' The first way of writing it limits me. It assumes that what is true now is true for evermore. It stops me from even thinking about the possibility of progress. It doesn't allow me to access my potential. So have another look at what you have written down, and see if you can turn some of your self-limiting 'Can'ts' around into more positive, and truer, statements.

Doing this exercise will also reveal your strengths and weaknesses. We are all gifted, but in different areas. You may be particularly good with elderly people, so putting yourself in situations where you meet them will give you lots of enjoyment, and confidence. If, on the other hand, you find it difficult to talk to them, accept it. Your strengths obviously lie in other areas which are equally valid, but different. If you were to put yourself in situations with them, unlike the other person, you would find your confidence in yourself ebbing away. Accept your strengths and build on them, but accept your weaknesses, too. If they are in an area which is important to you, then you can seek assistance to help you improve. If this area isn't important, then it doesn't matter. It's all right to be less than perfect at something. We all are. We're all human.

Likes and dislikes are also clues to knowing yourself. I particularly like cold weather. I love winter's wonderful frosty mornings when the air is crisp and the sun's shining in a beautiful blue sky. My heart sings on those mornings. Summer is my least favourite time. I find the heat too oppressive, I feel drained of energy and very uncomfortable. So in knowing this about myself (and it took a long time for me to admit it to sun-worshipping friends) I can plan holidays which are more in keeping with my likes and dislikes. And I know that if I were offered a job in the tropics I would be very unhappy if I accepted. My confidence would drain away as I struggled daily to cope with the extreme heat and humidity. I wouldn't be able to feel that I was coping well. Conversely, if I went to somewhere like Iceland, I would revel in the climate and feel quite confident about trekking through snow and ice. Wonderful. When you do what you enjoy, your confidence is bound to improve.

'People' also come into the likes and dislikes category. If loud, brash people are not your type, then admit it. If quiet, mousy types make you feel on edge, that's fine. It is written nowhere that you have to like everyone you meet or know. If someone you found charming at first now turns out to be an overwhelming drag, it is all right to admit that you would rather not be in their company.

Many of us are brought up to be nice to others. That's a noble virtue, but it can lead us into trouble if we misinterpret its meaning by becoming a doormat – which isn't good for your confidence. If you are uncomfortable with some people, it is fine for you to decide to call the friendship or relationship off. Otherwise your confidence will be affected as you try vainly to tame your own true self to fit in with others. It is your right to decide who you want to spend your valuable time with. You don't have to like everybody.

Situations are also open to likes and dislikes. Try to be honest with yourself about those you prefer to avoid. I must be careful here, because when you start to have panic attacks they can lead you to agoraphobic avoidance of places where you have had one. Avoiding a situation because you had a panic attack there is not what I am referring to. What I mean is that there are some situations which you may have disliked before you ever experienced a panic attack, but which you may not have had the confidence to own up to disliking.

Think about those situations. It is all right to admit that you find your friends' parties tiring affairs. They throw wild, all-night sessions, while you prefer a gin and tonic with a few close friends who can hear each other speak. Or vice versa. We don't have to like a situation just because it is expected of us/other people like it/you don't want to offend anyone by turning down the invitation. It really is much better to admit to other people (but yourself first) that there are some things you genuinely prefer to others. Make a list of the situations or places you like and dislike. Do be careful, though, not to include those which you now dislike only because you have had a panic attack there.

There may be some items on your list which all fall into the same category. For example, you may have put any social situation under the 'Dislike' heading. If this is the case, it might be worth getting to know yourself a little better and ask whether you would eventually like to be able to enjoy those situations. If so, you could consider what you might do to reach that point. There are many books available to help guide you through learning new social skills. There may also be courses available in your area. Contact your local citizen's advice bureau or library who may have a list. And remember that at this moment we have yet to realize our fullest potential. All of us are capable of handling ourselves well in any social situation. All of us. And when you can, then is a good time to decide which situations you enjoy more than others. You will then be choosing from a position of strength, in knowing what you like and why.

Once you start to know yourself better, you will begin to feel more self-confident. You will have the sense of being with a friend, rather than a stranger. Then, when you realize you are in a situation which you dislike, or are talking to someone who bores you, you will have the courage to say to yourself 'I don't like this. I'm going to go elsewhere instead, to somewhere I do like.' And when you do say that, it is OK. You have the absolute right to be true to yourself and do what you want to do. So do it.

Taking Positive Action

Learning how to say 'No' to others and 'Yes' to yourself is one of the most liberating things you can do for your confidence. When you say 'no' (when that is what you really want to say), you are establishing a more confident you. As someone who panics, you may be prone to listening to other people's problems and letting them make heavy demands on you and your time. But what happens to your own needs, and who listens to your problems? There comes a time when you have to start listening to your own voice.

You can begin practising saying 'no' by listening to the radio or watching TV and denying every single statement the presenter or newsreader makes – just for the hell of it. It can be good fun and it gets you used to challenging what you hear, not only from others but also from your own negative voices when they sound. Become used to having your voice heard, rather than mouthing an echo of what others say, or nodding quietly in agreement. Listen, as you assert your choice to be different.

Being able to live assertively really does help your confidence develop. Instead of being either a doormat or someone who reacts aggressively in stressful situations, assertiveness allows you to be yourself in a calm, assured way. If you think you would like to find out more about how to assert yourself, there are many good books around and possibly some courses at your local adult education centre. You can begin to assert yourself now by deciding to find out more, and doing some research into it. Asking for help is one of the most pro-active things you can do. Instead of waiting for another stressful situation to present itself, start to act now. Take the initiative and begin to find out how you can become more assertive. Your library is a good place to start.

In chapter 8 we talked about affirmations; positive statements about yourself which help re-program your thoughts, and therefore your actions. Affirmations can also be used to help you regain your self-confidence. Perhaps unconsciously, you have been giving yourself damaging, negative statements about your ability to cope, as a result of the panic attacks you have been experiencing. To counteract them, say affirmations which encourage a positive attitude about yourself. Here are some which you could use:

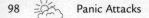

I love and accept myself.

I am confident in my own abilities.

I am capable and strong.

I am sure of myself.

I trust my own judgement.

I am positive about my life, my work, my relationships.

You may be able to think of some special ones for yourself. Remember that a thought is a thing and when you start to think these positive statements, they will start to work straight away. Saying 'I am' is now, in the present – and that is where we always are.

Affirmations will help your confidence build from the inside and support the new-found knowledge which you have about yourself. You can also start to be more kind to You. When you experience panic attacks it is all too easy to judge yourself too harshly. You may think how weak and stupid you were to go funny during that dinner party, or how awful you were to have an attack right in the middle of that man's speech. The truth is that you are not stupid or weak, and there is nothing awful about feeling unwell (for whatever reason) in the middle of anyone's speech. Reverse the roles; think about how you would react if you were the one up on the platform. You would probably be so concerned about keeping your place in your notes and not stumbling over words that someone leaving the room would not be of the slightest importance to you. If you saw someone else go a little pale at the dinner table, what would you think of them? You would wonder if they were feeling all right, and simply be concerned. What else do you think someone would think? What do you think others are saying to themselves when you have a panic attack? You may be surprised that the majority of them probably don't even notice. They're all too busy thinking about the impression they themselves are making to wonder about anyone else. This may help to remove another fear which you may have surrounding panic attacks – the fear of what others may think of you or how they might react if you should have one. At the end of the day, it doesn't matter what other people think because they will be far too engrossed in themselves. Stop worrying about them, and remind yourself of the confidence you have by saying your positive affirmations.

People who do lack confidence tend to have too high expectations of themselves. This may be true of you. So instead, try to speak to yourself with kindness, gentleness and understanding. If you feel too tired to keep that appointment this evening, that's fine. It's all right to be tired, and it's better in the long run to look after yourself by not overdoing things. So be proactive, cancel that appointment and fix another one for a time when you are less busy. Then go home and pamper yourself. Make your favourite meal and eat it watching a good film on television. Have a long bath, read while you're doing it or just let your mind wander into dreamtime. Then cuddle up with a hot water bottle, your partner or an enjoyable book, whatever makes you feel good. Treating yourself kindly recharges your batteries and helps you start the next day refreshed and knowing you can cope. And if, during the day, you have had a panic attack, be kind to yourself about that, too. Think instead about what you can learn from it. What led up to this one? Did you catch your thoughts in time? Having a panic attack isn't a failure; it's an experience which you can learn something from every time.

After completing the previous exercise about likes and dislikes, you may now have a list (written or in your head) of the people you prefer to be with. This is important, especially now as you start to rebuild your confidence. Negative people make others feel negative, too. Positive people give you energy, lift you, and can help you feel at ease. Surround yourself with as many of this sort as you can. Avoid the negative ones who will drag you down and sap your confidence. They are not the ones who will support and encourage you. Instead, seek out the positive ones who can. If they are close friends, confide in them about your feelings. Ask them for a bit of moral support, a bit of encouragement, for the time being. Tell them about how unsure you feel of yourself and that your confidence could do with a bit of bolstering up. Good friends and positive people will rally round, but they can't do it if they don't know about how you feel. There is more about friends and family in chapter 15.

Besides being positive to yourself, and surrounding yourself with positive people in situations you like, you can also be positive towards others. We all need encouragement, compliments and kind words, whether we have panic attacks or not. And when you start to put out positive energies you will find that you get more of the same coming back to you. Giving out to others has the strange effect of making you feel good, too. And anything which makes you feel good is bound to increase your confidence.

Self-confidence is a powerful ally in helping you bring your panic attacks to an end. In the next chapter we'll discover how you can start to exercise it to help prevent panic attacks occurring.

Summary

- ◆ It is understandable that your confidence may have taken a dip because of panic attacks. It will come back.
- ◆ Getting to know yourself will help you find it again.
- ◆ When you know what you like and dislike it is easier to be confident about yourself.
- ◆ Learning to be more assertive can help.
- ◆ Be pro-active and start to include as many positive elements in your life as you can.
- ◆ Be kind to yourself.

10

Positive Prevention

Back in chapter 5 we looked at the progressive cycle of panic attacks and how you can cue yourself into one, barely realizing it, once you have unconsciously received a signal which says 'threat'. In order to end panic attacks you have to break this cycle of repetition.

We have already looked at what panic attacks really are, to help remove fear of them. We've also looked at the positive impact your thoughts can have in turning negative cues into more positive reassurances. Your overall confidence provides the important framework for all this to take place, and we have looked at what you can do to improve this, too.

All these things can help weaken the vicious cycle of attacks. There is another way to bolster the effectiveness of the work you can do in those areas. It is time to consider what you can do at the initial stage, prior to having an attack and prior to feeling the effects of adrenalin release. What else can you do to help keep the levels of additional anxiety from rising beyond an acceptable level?

Coping Strategies

I mentioned earlier the difference between coping and curing. Coping is only a temporary measure, while curing offers long-term results because it addresses root causes.

There are a number of supports which people who panic develop in an attempt to find something which helps them cope, since curing probably hasn't even been mentioned. Personally, I see long-term medication in this light.

Drugs

In the short term, drugs may give the respite you need from the onslaught of attacks, and allow you to calm down enough to start addressing the problem in a more positive and pro-active way. They may have their place in the overall strategy, but there are three issues about depending on drugs as a long-term solution. One is that studies have not been able to prove conclusively that drugs are always a cure for panic attacks (and nor are they free from side effects); secondly, they do not address underlying issues, or attempt to get to the root causes (although, to be fair, if doctors assume there is a purely biological reason for panic attacks, prescribing medication is their way of addressing what they believe to be root causes); the third issue is that the way this form of treatment is given does not encourage you to take personal responsibility for yourself.

Medication is now being used by some doctors in conjunction with counselling or psychotherapy. This is a much better balance to aim for if you do choose to accept drugs as part of your treatment. That particular choice is up to you, after discussing it at length with your doctor and weighing up all the pros and cons. Combining it with some supportive work may not only help increase the effectiveness of the medication, but also help you discover one or two answers for yourself.

'Props'

Some people who have been prescribed tranquillizers or another type of drug say they don't necessarily take them when they should, but instead carry one around with them in their pocket or purse 'just in case', like Brian who said that it helped him having the 'knowledge that I can always take a pill if I have to, although I don't need them at present.' Others adopt a similar attitude and take reassurance from having a small bottle of water with them or a packet of mints, like Melanie who always used to carry them with her wherever she went in case her mouth went dry, which was part of her cue for an attack. Having a sip of water or a mint helped her ward it off.

There is obviously nothing wrong with having props to help you through, but props are not the answer. If you think they are, you could be in trouble when, one day, you suddenly find they fail you. The effect could be a real blow if you have put your absolute faith in them without developing other more pro-active strategies which work toward a more long-term answer. Relying on props such as these keeps you at a distance from learning how to rely on yourself.

Alcohol

Alcohol is another prop which many people frequently turn to, even those who don't experience panic attacks. Feelings of intimidation or extreme discomfort in social situations appear to be ameliorated by one or two drinks. Depending on them to see you through is again only a temporary coping mechanism and one which cannot lead to a cure. Indeed, it can bring further problems in its wake if the dependency escalates – drinking before the event, and then afterwards because your body has itself become dependent on the alcohol.

There is a link between panic attacks and alcohol abuse. Whether the panic attacks begin first and alcohol is used in an attempt at self-treatment, or whether drinking excessively causes attacks is unclear. Whichever is true, alcohol is a prop which offers no cure for panic attacks and can lead to real problems; possibly alcoholism. If you drink to ward off attacks, a better approach would be to ask yourself why you feel uncomfortable in such situations. When you understand why, you can then start to work out what to do about it. Learning how to assert yourself could be the answer, or developing your confidence in social settings. There are many books available from your local library which can help.

Avoidance

Avoiding situations is also a common way for people to cope with the threat of panic attacks. This is understandable, but it cannot possibly help you in the long term. Repeatedly leaving situations only serves to encourage you to do the same again next time, denying yourself a valuable learning experience; an opportunity to practise by trial and error. Without any attempt at dealing with the situation, you remove the chance of succeeding in it.

When you choose to escape from a situation you take your feelings with you, because they are there inside you and not in the meeting, the church or the bus queue. They don't go away as soon as you set foot outside, so you could just as well stay where you are and let the feelings subside as you know they will. You now know that you will come to no harm, that you will not lose control or faint or go mad. And learning to accept the wave of sensations while you stay put is one very positive step forward. Leaving the situation is negative and does nothing to help you move ahead.

Continually turning away, as chapter 5 explained, can lead to extremes of avoidance. Eventually you can become so convinced that you will have an attack there (wherever 'there' is) that you decide to avoid it all together. The long-term result is that you can then become so lacking in confidence, and unable to cope with what has become a strange situation to you, that it only serves to worsen your position.

However, leaving an uncomfortable situation is tempting. Next time, if you really do feel that you have to go, see if you can hang on for just a few more seconds, then a few more, and just another. Remind yourself that, of course, you can leave at any moment you choose to. No one is stopping you. But see if you can sit or stand for just one more second. Then if you do leave, do so in as positive a frame of mind as you can and with determination. Instead of 'I've got to get out of here!' think 'I've stayed as long as I feel I can. Now I choose to leave.' And above all, do try to return straight away, as soon as you feel calm again. You know what they say about falling off a horse: that you should get back on it straight away before you have time even to think about it. The same is also true here. Go straight back in and remind yourself that you can leave again if you need to, but that you probably won't now that the attack is over.

If avoidance has become a real problem for you, your doctor may suggest desensitization through behaviour therapy, described in chapter 6. This can work with some people, but again, I feel that it does not address underlying issues. 'Getting used to' is not the same as 'accepting'. It implies a defensive stance, a brick wall of will power. Walls can be breached and only serve to dam the tide of feelings and emotions temporarily. However, like medication, behaviour therapy can be of use to some people and help as part of an overall strategy. It could be a therapy which you choose as a useful tool to have. Personally, I'm not convinced that it is a cure for panic attacks, although it does help a lot of people cope.

Back To You

So if these coping mechanisms are not the answer, what is? The answer, as you may have guessed already, is echoed again in the Delphic 'Know Thyself'. Without self-knowledge you are sure to be at a loss as to how to take more positive action. You need to know what you are about so that you can then act accordingly. When you know what your strengths and weaknesses are, you can tailor your life to enhance the one and develop strategies to improve the other. Without that knowledge you are adrift on a sea of unknowing without a rudder in sight, not realizing that the captain is yourself. If you need to, go back to chapter 9 and read again about starting to learn about yourself.

Besides using our natural abilities, we also act according to sets of internal rules. If they are in accord with us then we stay in harmony. If they aren't, they can cause lots of additional stress. These rules consist of our attitudes, beliefs, and concepts. None of these were there when we were born. They have all developed under the influence of what we can call 'significant others': parents, siblings, friends, colleagues, religion, culture and society at large. Unfortunately, some of the things we believe are not necessarily true. For example, you may believe you are useless. That is not true. I know it is untrue because of the untapped potential which you have. And special though you are, it is highly unlikely that you are the first human being ever to be without potential, and therefore useless! However, that message could have been one which your parents gave you when you were too young to realize that what they said was not a universal truth, and that they could be wrong. Similarly, peer group pressure can lead us to adopt the attitude that it is unacceptable to ask for help or to show kindness to others.

Other examples of unhelpful rules are those which tell you that you 'must', 'should' or 'can't'. These words sound as though they are already written in stone for evermore. They aren't. But that is how we tend to see them and apply each one with a broad sweep across too many areas of our lives. Again, the words were taught to us when we were young and probably without being given a qualifying proviso of when they were appropriate. So now we use them all the time to apply to everything. We feel we 'can't' do lots of things, even though our inner voice is saying 'Yes, I want to go for it.'

We all need some rules by which to live, but you may have been living with the same ones for too long; the ones which belonged to your parents, teachers or friends of long ago. Now is a good time to start having a look at some of the beliefs, attitudes and concepts you have, and weed out those which are now inappropriate so that you can adopt more flexible ones, in line with the true self you are beginning to know.

Watch out for all those 'shoulds', 'musts' and 'can'ts'. Listen out for the negative and self-limiting concepts which you have about yourself, and the beliefs which cause you internal stress and strain. Adapting them will help reduce that anxiety level of yours, which is probably too high even now.

Here are some examples with alternatives:

I can't paint.

I really enjoy using paints and creating my own images in the colours I like.

I must always put other people's needs first.

My needs are just as important as other people's.

I should be doing better.

I have achieved a lot so far. I am doing as well as I can right now.

Or: *I could do better, but I choose to go at this comfortable pace.*

I must be useless if I can't do that.

I'm finding it difficult to do that, but I am still a person of worth.

I should accept my lot in life and be grateful.

This situation is not to my liking. To change it I can seek outside help/express my feelings about it/devise a plan of action.

I must not lose my temper.

Occasionally losing my temper is only human, and is sometimes the most appropriate form of action.

Emotions and feelings can also cause internal stress when they are blocked and frustrated in their attempts to be let out. This could be due to another belief that we 'can't' show affection or anger. Bottling up powerful emotions causes difficulties, not only within ourselves but also with relationships. Communicating how we feel is vitally important if we are to live our lives authentically. Assertiveness training can help, and may be a tool which you could use in your strategy of positive prevention of attacks. Removing communication blocks removes additional stress.

There may be emotions which are buried deep in the past, or there may be inner conflicts which remain unresolved. We need to understand, respect and accept even difficult feelings if we are to progress. Controlling our emotions, or being controlled by them, creates imbalance. Living in harmony with them is what we can aim for, but to do that we need to know what they are. Accessing these emotions can be difficult. But if you want to break that cycle of panic attacks and you know that unresolved issues are creating problems for you, then you could decide to take pro-active measures and ask your doctor for details of counsellors, therapists or self-help groups which might be of help. This is a very positive way forward and some people may be able to get a direct referral.

Raising your awareness of what is going on inside can be echoed by also becoming aware, in a non-panic state, of what your body is telling you. It seems quite odd that on the one hand you are highly sensitive to bodily sensations, ready to interpret any as a possible panic, while on the other you are unaware of the mounting stresses and strains leading up to an escalation of anxiety.

We tend to be brought up in a state of ignorance about our bodies. Instead of being taught how to listen to them, we ignore signals they send out until illness or disease becomes their last resort in trying to tell us that all is not well. But before we reach that point, the body will have switched on a few red warning lights in an attempt to warn either of problems inside us, or disturbing elements in our environment. However, we tend not to notice these warning lights, and fail to recognize signs of stress at an early stage.

Without this bodily self-knowledge we're going to find ourselves in difficulties. Headaches go unheeded or are treated with a pill to stop them; skin rashes are seen as bothersome but no more; stomach upsets are given antacids or X-rays. Instead of looking at why we may be experiencing them we think only of how to get rid of symptoms. A little enlightenment beforehand could help us recognize danger signals before they develop into real problems.

This applies to high anxiety and stress levels, precursors to panic. We go through each day, concentrating on our tasks and chores, giving only a cursory thought to our hard-working bodies. We feed them, clothe and wash them, but leave the rest to chance. Aches and pains are seen as a nuisance, not as helpful indicators. Wherever you are right now, turn your attention to your face – are you looking calm and serene or are you frowning, tight-lipped or clenching your jaw? Where are your shoulders? Are they relaxed, or tensed into a position up around your ears somewhere? Which way is your neck pointing? Up and down your back as it should be, or is it tensed into a thrust forward position? Are your shoulders on either side of your chest or are they trying desperately to meet in front of your very eyes? And how are your stomach muscles? They may be less than firm but still be clenched in tension.

Scanning your body and putting even those few points to right can have an instant effect. Feeling more relaxed in your body helps your mind relax. Regularly doing this simple exercise is a good preventative measure. Try to get into the habit of doing it a few times a day. Notice the tension in your muscles and relax them down. It only takes a few seconds to do but can be of enormous help.

Breathing incorrectly is an important indicator of stress. It's been mentioned already that hyperventilating has been linked with the onset of panic attacks. Being aware of doing it and changing your breathing pattern can be a great step towards positive prevention. Poor breathing habits easily develop but are just as easy to correct.

Place one hand on your upper chest and one just above your navel. As you breathe, notice which hand moves. It should be the one on your stomach. If it isn't, you are breathing incorrectly and possibly hyperventilating. Breathing should make your stomach move in and out as your diaphragm expands and contracts, to draw air in and out of your lungs. So, keep the hand on your upper chest still, and make your stomach move in and out instead. Practise breathing slowly and calmly in this way, then check throughout the day whether you are still doing it correctly.

There are other signals which our bodies send out. Tiredness, fatigue and irritability are also red light danger signs. Learn what your tolerance thresholds are and respond to them. If you begin to feel tired, go and rest. If you start to feel irritable, you need a break for a while. Fatigue can't be combated by doing more work. Pushing our bodies, ignoring these danger signals, is a recipe for disaster for anyone, and a sure bet for a panic attack for you. Your body will take over in an attempt to protect you and do what it knows best: to get ready to fight or take flight from a situation which is adding even more stress to your already overloaded system.

Positive Action

Knowing and understanding your body's needs for rest, relaxation and recuperation is already a positive step towards panic prevention. Once you become more aware, you can begin to plan pro-active ways to support and reinforce.

We've already mentioned relaxation and breathing correctly. These sorts of exercises are useful tools to have in your prevention kit. They are much better ones than carrying a tablet or packet of mints around with you, because they teach you how to rely on yourself. Drugs may calm you down, but so can you.

Relaxing can pose a threat to some people who panic; it can provoke an attack. This apparent contradiction can seem mystifying, but not if you understand that tension can be used as a defence against unwelcome thoughts and feelings. For some people, letting that tension go can feel like opening the flood gates. Without understanding this, it can be most distressing. There you are trying to take positive action, and it appears to have the opposite effect. If this happens to you, try to go with it. Listen to those voices within you. Ignoring them can't possibly help. Listen to what they have been trying to tell you and acknowledge them. If you find this too difficult to do alone, a supportive friend or relative might be able to help. I know that sometimes people feel uncomfortable talking to those they know well about difficult, personal issues, so finding a counsellor or therapist might be the answer. Taking time to talk out your inner fears and worries is an excellent preventative measure. We all need to let off steam and talk through problems with someone. Therapists and counsellors provide the supportive environment you need to be able to do this with confidence. Have a word with your doctor for recommendations, or contact your local MIND group who should have lists of local people who can help.

Knowing your body better, you can now respond positively to tiredness or anxiety. Take yourself off for five minutes, five hours or five days; whatever it needs to rebalance you and recharge those worn batteries. Working on regardless may seem noble and tough, but when you know it could lead to a panic attack it is sheer foolhardiness. No doubt you will now jump up and down and shriek that you couldn't possible take time out (even for five minutes). Yes, sometimes it is difficult to come to a sudden halt and it may cause more practical problems as a result – unless you take pro-active measures. Now might be a good time to acquire some new practical skills to help you do that.

For example, do you use your time efficiently? Are you able to delegate, or do you think that only you can be trusted to do things properly (another rigid, outdated rule)? How well do you tackle problems? Do you approach them systematically or do you let them run around unchecked inside your head? Top managers have these skills as part of their management repertoire. If they can help multinational companies run efficiently, they could also help you run your life better.

Time management helps you work efficiently and plan for productive rest periods (studies show that all work and no play not only makes you dull but drastically decreases work efficiency). It is a good way to make sure you take those much-needed regular breaks which alleviate rising tension and anxiety levels.

Delegation takes away pressure. It can also motivate others, including family members and friends as well as work colleagues. Calling house meetings to discuss and agree on delegation of tasks (and penalties) productively shifts unwieldy workloads from your shoulders. You'll be happier, and so will everyone else when they see how much less irritable you are.

Problem-solving techniques are also easily learned. Unresolved problems create worry; worry creates anxiety, and anxiety can lead to panic attacks. Solve the problem and you kill the worry; kill the worry and you reduce the possibility of another attack. It's so easy to let the mind run around seemingly endless problems, but by learning to take hold of each in turn and deal with them appropriately, you come one step nearer to positively preventing an attack.

Going into difficult situations can easily lead to worry about whether you will have a panic or not. You now know how to help by using your thoughts in a positive way. You can also pre-plan positive strategies. Whatever the situation, plan to build relaxing breaks into it. If it is a party, visit the bathroom regularly or step outside to inspect the garden for a breather. If you realize the root of the problem is boredom, then leave decisively. At the cinema, sit in an aisle seat and plan ahead to have one or two breaks, before you have a chance to start feeling panicky. There are few situations for which you cannot plan a strategy. Even meetings can have breaks included. You can easily excuse yourself for a moment – setting your watch bleeper for a convenient time is one possible strategy. Then you will not have to resort to 'escaping' on the verge of panic.

Taking positive preventative action not only helps to ward off possible attacks, but also reminds you that you are in control. As a result your confidence increases and a light at the end of the tunnel slowly starts to come into view.

In the next chapter we'll have a close look into your lifestyle and how that can help or hinder you.

Summary

◆ Depending on coping mechanisms will not cure.
◆ Knowing yourself and your body will.
◆ Have a look at your personal rules. Update any which no longer apply or which hold you back from being your true self.
◆ Start to plan those positive prevention strategies which will help you – now. Take a few minutes to write a list before you go on to the next chapter. For example, planning for short breaks next time you are in a meeting, or finding out about assertiveness training.

11

Your Lifestyle

In chapter 3 we looked at how panic attacks can affect your life, and you may have had to make many changes to 'accommodate' them into yours. But the relationship between panic attacks and lifestyle works the other way too. The sort of life you lead may have some bearing on them. I can see that this was the case for me, when I now look back to the time when they started to happen.

I've already mentioned the major changes which were happening at the time: buying my first flat, my mother dying soon after, splitting up with my boyfriend, and gaining promotion to work in a place where I wasn't particularly happy. Those major changes underpinned the way I began to run my life. I had moved to a completely new area which had no real focal point, and I felt a certain sense of isolation. Although I had moved nearer to work and where most of my friends lived, the flat wasn't easy to get to and from. I took a certain amount of refuge in work and spent more time there than strictly necessary, and then developed the habit of going for a drink after work with colleagues. By the time I came home I was exhausted from the strains and pressures of the new job, working extra hours, and drinking after work. My diet relied too heavily on take-aways or instant-type meals which were more convenient for the life I was leading. I was certainly too tired to think of cooking gourmet meals when I went home.

Socializing with friends took a back seat, crammed into weekends along with shopping and other domestic chores which I never managed to do during the week. It became too easy not to bother making any arrangements; sleep seemed more important.

Gradually I was becoming more stressed and strained until I felt that I was on a roundabout which was getting out of control. It was making me giddy, and I could barely keep up with the pace of things. Something had to give. It was me. My first panic attack struck. But looking back, how could I possibly have thought it was 'out of the blue'?

Other people report similarly trying lifestyles during their episodes of panic attacks. Jenny says 'Then, I was a very highly strung person. Now I take it all in my stride.' Melanie compares then and now: 'Now I'm totally independent. I'm totally in control of my life in comparison with then. I was living through my partner. I didn't have a career then and I wasn't financially independent. Emotionally I'm in control in comparison, too. I'm the dominant person now and others rely on me instead of the other way round.' 'Boredom. Non-activity. I did nothing,' was how yet another person described his unsatisfactory lifestyle at the time.

Your lifestyle may not be the cause of panic attacks, but an unsatisfactory one can lead to unnecessary stress on an already overloaded system. So let's have a look at yours. Just as you must know yourself to be able to change things, knowing your own lifestyle is a prerequisite for improving it.

Your Current Lifestyle

As happened with me, it is all too easy to become caught up in your life and not realize where it is all leading. You lurch from one week to the next, unable to see anything clearly except the odd birthday or celebration as it flashes quickly past, and then it's back on that roundabout again. On the other hand, your problem could be days which drag slowly by. With little excitement and no busy routine, perhaps you feel quite jealous of the hectic pace with which others struggle to cope. The truth is that neither is appropriate if they throw you out of balance and leave you with a feeling of disharmony. Too little structure in the day can be as stressful as too much.

Try to be as honest as you can with yourself in thinking about your own lifestyle. Hiding from the truth only keeps things as they are and prevents you from moving forward to better times. We talked before about the potential we all have as human beings. By extension, this also applies to our lives in general. We can have so much better ones, if only we realize.

Home

To begin with, think about your home life. It should be a source of joy, a refuge from the demanding outside world, a place you look forward to going back to when you are away. I wonder if you think of your home in that way. Do you really like the way your home looks, how it feels, where it is, the neighbours, the town you live in? It needn't be a palace, nor be expensively decorated, so long as it gives you pleasure and contentment. Living in an environment which causes you distress is harmful. Flinching because of the appalling decor every time you walk into your living room is hardly conducive to helping you live a stress-free life. Make a list of the things which affect you and you would like to change.

What about relationships within your home? They should also be a source of love, joy, support and comfort. Family life can be exciting, challenging, and fulfilling. It can also be the opposite. Perhaps there is a persistent bone of contention within the family, or maybe a lack of understanding has developed as members begin to change and mature. There are always ups and downs in the life of every family but when they become the norm, stress and anxiety levels for everyone can become unbearable and explosive. Instead of home being a sanctuary, it becomes a thing to dread and a prison in itself. What would you like to improve about your relationships with the people you live with?

Work

Our jobs of work are important in the sense of purpose they give us. Studies show a clear link between type of occupation and job satisfaction.

Those who work in jobs which offer no sense of responsibility, and where people feel a lack of personal control over what they do, tend to give least satisfaction. Production line workers would fall into this category. However, those who work in small companies where it is easier to have a sense of responsibility about what you do, even though they may have to work longer hours, tend to have the greatest job satisfaction. So too do executives who benefit from the sense of control which they experience in their positions.

The type of work you do may be important, but so too are the relationships at your place of work. Whether you have a difficult journey to get there may also affect your enjoyment. Future prospects may be a concern for you, too. Many people worry about the possibility of redundancy – an efficient anxiety provoker. And the strain of being unemployed long term goes without saying. Make a list of the things about your work life which you would like to change for the better.

Responsibilities

The number and type of responsibilities and commitments you have can affect your sense of well-being. Feeling crushed by too many can leave you feeling unable to cope with other stresses and strains. Have a look at the ones you have. You may have acquired too many over the years and now is a good time to have a more objective look at them all. For example, a handful of local groups with which you're involved could each have earmarked you again for numerous activities throughout the year, while you're already floundering with appearing to be the one person solely responsible for the family finances/shopping/cleaning. Perhaps there are some activities you could share, others you could shrug off, one or two you could reschedule.

Money

Money can also be a source of stress; normally when there isn't enough, but different spending priorities between partners can also cause problems. One partner wants to save and go on holiday, while the other prefers to have a good time at the pub – now. Conflicts like this can be incredibly stressful, as can poor money management skills.

Diet

What is your diet like? We are what we eat and if you live on irregular, poorly-balanced meals your body will struggle to work efficiently. This was one important aspect when my attacks started; it was so easy to slip into unhealthy eating habits. Recently I was asked to take part in a Government food survey and write down everything I ate for a whole week. What a revelation it was. Although I now consider myself to be conscientious about diet, I could see from the diary that there is still room for improvement. Do the same and keep a food diary for a week. You may be equally surprised. Our selective memories quietly forget those cakes, biscuits and odd glasses of wine.

Low Blood Sugar

It is worth mentioning here about the effect of eating too many sugar-rich foods on blood sugar levels. Without going into too many details, when you eat large amounts of these foods your body releases equally large amounts of insulin to cope with the influx. It works incredibly efficiently in reducing the amount of sugar in your blood, but continues to have its effect some time afterwards and leads to a further reduction. The result is low blood sugar, even though you ate a significant amount. People think the answer is to eat more sweet things, but that only sets the swing off again. The answer is to eat less sugar and let your body find its natural, balanced level.

The symptoms of low blood sugar include light-headedness, sweating, shaking, palpitations and others. You'll see the similarity between these and panic attack symptoms; someone who temporarily has low blood sugar can misinterpret the shaking as the start of another attack, and give themselves the incorrect mental cue. This is another reason to have a good look at your diet to see if you too eat more sugar than necessary.

Your Own Needs

And where are you in all this? How do you spend your leisure and pleasure time? Think about the enjoyment you have in life. Or do you feel that all your time is spent in giving pleasure to others and seeing to their needs? What about your own? Each time you deny your own needs, you deny your life. Denying your life leads to feelings of hopelessness. Take a look at the way your needs are met and the things which give you positive, enjoyable feelings.

There are other things which contribute to our lifestyles. Wider economic, social and political pressures all affect us in one way or another. The emphasis and relationship between all the different factors changes for each and every one of us. What you need to do is isolate those issues which are out of balance and having a negative effect on you. They could be the very things which keep the scales tipped too near the point of panic in your life. You are at a time in your life where a supportive, enjoyable, harmonious lifestyle is a necessity. By looking at what yours is like and the things which affect it, you can begin to turn it into what you need.

Secondary Gains

Panic attacks are unpleasant. For some people, though, they subconsciously offer a way of dealing with other issues. Think about whether this applies to you. Panic attacks may be a way out of a situation which you don't like, such as shopping chores or a job you loathe. They can provide you with a good excuse for not daring to test yourself at work for fear of failure. They can also provide a means of redressing imbalances in relationships, making your partner notice you, bonding you closer together.

This by no means applies to everyone, but do try to be honest with yourself if you think it may be true for you. When you can admit to those secondary gains which you receive as a by-product from having panic attacks, you are then in a position to start taking positive action to tackle any underlying issues instead of putting yourself through such painful experiences with each panic attack you have.

Deciding to Change

It is often said that we are creatures of habit. Some of us would rather stick with the familiar unpleasantness we know rather than risk a change to the unfamiliar. No matter how comforting that familiarity may appear, if your lifestyle gives you less joy than you need, it will make it harder for you to bring your panic attacks to an end. You may find it useful to re-read the chapters about personal power (chapter 7) and confidence (chapter 9) at this point. Practise those affirmations. Realizing you have the power and using it to build your confidence will help you address those lifestyle elements which could do with a good shake-up.

Deciding to change your lifestyle is your responsibility. In the last chapter we talked about learning new problem-solving skills. Now is a good time to put them into action. Define any problem areas in your life, look at possible solutions, draw up a plan of action. Some things cannot be changed, in which case you can change your own attitude towards it, reject the thing in question, or simply accept it. Accepting positively is different from putting up with in resentment, or giving in through weakness. It is a positive action and sometimes the most sensible solution.

Change can also bring stress in its own wake. People who panic are vulnerable to the effects of major change, so do think carefully about any you might now be thinking of making. Although you may have made decisions about changes you want to make, it is also sensible to decide when you want them to take place. Setting the change for some time in the near future, rather than immediately, could give you the time to make plans without creating the stress of rushing through. It allows you to become accustomed to wielding your personal power and taking control of your life. You are not in a race, so set your own easy pace and timetable of events. Knowing you are going to make changes to your life could be the motivation you have been looking for to learn how to stop your panic attacks once and for all. Take the time to plan and find the outside help (perhaps professional) you may need to help you achieve your goals.

Some Suggestions

In chapter 4 we looked at some 'Agents Provocateurs'. Have another look at that list (page 48) and see if there are any in your life which you could eliminate. As you get to know yourself and your life better, you may find others which also raise your anxiety and stress levels too high, and each panic attack from now on is an opportunity to learn even more – about them and yourself. Karen has the right attitude. She is the one who sees her panic attacks as being a huge and welcome kick up the backside, and now thinks herself lucky to have had them, so sharply did they make her focus on the disharmony in her life. Like her, you can use this period in your life to begin to tune into your finer sensitivities which have somehow become dulled in our quest for more money, more power, more possessions, more, more, more.

We are led to believe that we cannot be happy unless we follow that acquisitive path, for which you need more and more money. But there are lots of things in life which are free or very cheap and which really do feed the soul. Music can calm and revive and play an important part in helping to reduce anxiety. Colour cheers the spirit, or again can calm you down – some prison cells, used to hold particularly violent or aggressive people, are painted bubble-gum pink for this reason. It works. Wearing your favourite colours and surrounding yourself with ones you like can also have a positive effect on your mood and sense of well-being.

Pleasant smells always cheer me up. The smell of freshly cut grass, or earth after a summer rainfall almost send me into ecstasies, as do freshly baked bread, fresh coffee and sizzling bacon. Some of those are free, others cost only pennies (making your own bread can save some). Breathing fresh air always makes me feel much better, too.

Working at my desk, I sometimes forget how many hours I spend without getting outside at all – I've still a lot to learn about looking after myself and giving myself even more good experiences.

Clean bed sheets, hot baths, good books, laughter and my cat are important positives in my life. They are easy to take for granted or overlook, but now that I have woken up to myself a little more, I can appreciate those things and make sure they are integrated into my life on a regular basis to cheer, calm or recharge. Think about those things which particularly give you pleasure. They may be some of those same things I enjoy. Whatever they are, make sure you now include as many as you can, as regularly as you need to.

I mentioned relaxation in the last chapter, but it will do no harm to mention it again. We can too easily press through each day only to collapse exhausted into our beds at night, even then without being fully relaxed. This used to be the case with me. A few seconds' relaxation throughout the day can really help keep those anxiety levels down. Imagine you have been carrying two huge weights around, one in each hand, then let them go. This is a quick way to get you into a more relaxed pose, but deep relaxation may help further. Contact your local adult education institute to see if they run any classes there, or your GP may know of some. S/he may also be able to recommend a meditation class. These can be very helpful in learning how to calm mind and body into deep relaxation.

Exercise isn't everyone's idea of fun, but even I have to admit it is important in helping our bodies stay in good working order and reduce stress levels. Competitive sport could be counterproductive, but gentle movements such as in yoga may be more suitable and less stressful on your delicately balanced system, especially since exercise can provoke attacks in some people, so go easy. If you can handle more vigorous exercise, it will help burn off excess adrenalin and other anxiety-related biochemical residues. Exercise not only invigorates but also calms and improves your sense of well-being. Think about the benefits that a regular exercise routine could bring into your lifestyle.

After looking at your diet, you may have decided there is room for improvement. Besides avoiding sugary foods, increase your intake of fresh vegetables, wholemeal foods and fruit. Cut down on meat, and replace it with fish if you can't give up animal protein altogether.

When our bodies are under stress we use up our stores of vitamins more rapidly. Vitamin B complex is beneficial to the nerves and vitamin C is useful to help combat stress. Calcium has a calming effect. You may want to consider taking additional supplements of all three to make sure your supplies don't become too depleted, making your job that much harder as you start to take control over your panic attacks. There are many good books around which explain about vitamins and recommended dosages. Take a trip to your local library to find out more. Although there appears to be a wide range of differing attitudes about how much to take for a remedial or maintenance dose, at least there is agreement that vitamins are vitally important in helping our bodies function at their optimum levels.

Another dimension can be added to your life through helping others. Not the moaning friends who enjoy nagging about their latest problem; I mean those people who really are less fortunate than yourself. It's an odd thing that helping others can lead you to helping yourself. A shift of focus away from self-interests can help relieve your own worries and put them in a different perspective, but only get involved if you feel you could happily cope with the demands.

Other things you may like to consider including in your new lifestyle are activities which can positively help you live a more fulfilling life. Taking classes in communication skills, management, assertiveness or life skills can be a real help. But so can joining in sculpture classes, for example, if that's what you've always wanted to try. Now is the time to explore all those avenues which can lead you to a more enjoyable lifestyle.

Your Ideal Dream

What is your ideal dream of a life like? Where do you live and what do you do there? It doesn't matter whether it is practical or attainable at the moment, just acknowledge to yourself, out loud, what your dream really is. If you're lucky you may already have it, but in that case it's unlikely that you have been experiencing panic attacks and are reading this book. If not, what images come into your mind? For some it might be running for President, for others it might be deep-sea diving, while someone else can see themselves living in the countryside, far away from their present city life.

It is important to acknowledge what your dream is; otherwise, as the song goes, how are you going to make your dream come true? Knowing what your ideal is makes it easier to set your sights. And even if you can't reach your target, you will at least then be aiming in the right direction and be on your true path. If you really want to be an astronaut you will feel frustrated (perhaps without realizing why) if you choose to ignore your dream and go for a money-making job in finance. So you might be too old to go into space, but you could work in an allied field which keeps you in contact with your dream and on your chosen path. When you're on that path you can't go wrong. You're in tune with the real You. When Carlos Castaneda asked the Yaqui Indian which was the right path in life, he replied that the right path is the path with a heart. I cannot for one moment believe that the path can be right for anyone if it leads them to experiencing panic attacks.

Is your present path the one with a heart?

Summary

- Panic attacks can affect your life, but your lifestyle can also affect your panic attacks.
- Spend some time finding out where there's room for improvement in yours.
- Work out what you'd like to change and how. Ask friends or professionals for help if you need it.
- It's your responsibility how satisfying your lifestyle is. You can make it as bad or as good as you like.
- Find out what other pleasures you can include in your life.
- Acknowledge what your ideal dream of a life really is.
- Discover your own 'path with a heart'.

12

Complementary Therapies

Previously we looked at 'traditional' solutions to panic attacks, and their strengths and weaknesses. We then began to consider the role you play in your attacks, and how you can make use of your own considerable power to help bring them to an end – and improve your quality of life. Part of what has been suggested has aimed to empower you; to encourage you to accept full responsibility for what happens to you and realize the amount of control you do have.

The message is: you can do it. I know you can, because everyone (including you) has that vast reservoir of as-yet-untapped potential which I keep talking about. I know you can do it. However, you may recognize that you could do with some additional constructive help. Not in the form of prescriptions or unsatisfactory visits to your doctor, but something more useful. It's fine to acknowledge your need for that help. In making that acknowledgement you give yourself the option to do something positive.

Your doctor may be able to suggest some forms of help, such as local support groups. It can be an enormous relief to talk to people who have experienced the same things you have. S/he may also direct you to your local MIND group or to No Panic, both of which can offer valuable support. If you would like psychotherapeutic or counselling help, the doctor should be able to give you a referral or information about where you can find that sort of help. If you have family or lifestyle changes to make which you would like assistance with, s/he could point you in the right direction for this, too (for example, marriage guidance, bereavement support, child guidance, social services). You may not want to accept the prescription your doctor offers, but s/he can still be a useful source of other forms of help. Do ask. You have a right to that support. But if your doctor is particularly unhelpful, contact your local area health authority for the information you need. Their number will be in the telephone directory, or your local library should have it.

In this chapter we'll have a look at another area which could offer more of that valuable support you're looking for, but which your doctor is unlikely to be able to give you much information about: complementary therapies. Many people are starting to question the safety and wisdom of allopathic medicine (your doctor's sort), and are beginning to look for alternatives. With this growing awareness, complementary therapies are becoming more widely accepted, especially homoeopathy which is now available in Britain through the NHS.

Some sections of the medical profession are waking up to this and starting to realize the need to consider the whole mind/body of a person in planning any treatment (as complementary therapists do), rather than addressing just the symptoms. Although total acceptance by the medical establishment is a long way off yet, complementary therapies are available for you to consider now, and could provide useful additional tools for you to include in your panic attack prevention kit. There are a vast number of different types available, some of which may be useful for panic attacks.

How Complementary Therapies Could Help

Complementary therapies may be useful to people who panic in a number of ways, primarily in helping to reduce anxiety levels which appear to be an integral part of attacks.

Therapies could be described as falling into two main categories; those which address your mind and the thoughts you may have (this was dealt with in chapter 8), and those which treat your body. Having said this, mind and body are so closely interlinked that one inevitably affects the other. A therapy might be directed at either your thoughts or your physical sensations, but will probably end up affecting the other. Or you might want a therapy which will help you acquire new skills to be of direct use in learning how to stay calm, control your thoughts, be more assertive, reduce the frequency of attacks, or help you to cope with them better.

Complementary therapies can be incredibly enjoyable – a positive ingredient to include if you're aiming to improve the quality of your lifestyle. They can also increase your sense of well-being and have a very positive effect on those vitally important feelings of self-confidence which were discussed in chapter 9.

Which Therapy?

This question is really for you to answer. It is your decision. Since there is little comparative literature to support one therapy over another, it is your responsibility to investigate the possibilities and decide for yourself. We are all individual and we all have different needs. A therapy which is ideal for me may not provide what you want.

From the things you have started to find out about yourself, you may now be in a position to know that you would appreciate some help with sorting out what goes on in your head. You may have discovered some unresolved conflicts from your past which you feel are holding back your progress and having a negative effect on your life. Or you may now feel that you would like to know more about self-control and the power of thought, in which case you would be wise to look at those therapies which are more concerned with the mind.

Alternatively, you may be aware of how tense and unyielding your body has become through the effects of anxiety and constant worry about your next panic attack. Although you know your mind could do with a bit of work on it too, your priority might be to bring some respite from tension to your body. That's fine. It's up to you where you decide to start from, and finding a therapy which treats your body may bring enormous benefits to you and be what you need first.

In choosing a therapy there are other aspects to consider, such as whether you want individual treatment or group work. Price might be an important factor. Decide if you need to find someone local, or even someone who can visit you at home. Do you need to find a therapist who can do weekend or evening work? What do you need the therapy to help you achieve? What are your aims for going there? It might be something as vague as wanting to get more in touch with yourself. That's fine. So long as you know what you need, then it will make it easier to find a therapy which suits. You might be able to think of more things which are important to you and which may affect your final decision. Spend some time thinking about what other needs you have.

There are many books available on the wide range of different therapies. Take the initiative and make a trip to your local library; ask them for a reference book on complementary therapies. One which outlines a variety will be of most use to begin with, to help you compare without having to go into too much detail. Once you have identified those which you think might be able to offer what you are looking for, you can then do more specific in-depth reading.

How to Find a Therapist

Personal recommendation is one of the best ways of finding a therapist. Mention to friends and colleagues what you're interested in, and you may be surprised to find they have tried it/are using it/know of someone who does it/know of someone who has used it. It can make your research so much easier, but do remember that we all have our personal preferences, and what is wrong for someone else may not necessarily be inappropriate for you. If they went to a herbalist to help them give up smoking, they may have been disappointed with the results. However, it could be just what you need. Horses for courses. So weigh people's comments carefully.

Health food shops often have notice boards with advertisements for classes and therapists. If your local shop doesn't, suggest they

start one up. Some of the health magazines they sell advertise therapists, although they may be some distance from where you live. Still,
they could be worth looking into. Local papers also occasionally carry
advertisements, but use your judgement – the sort of massage you
want is probably not the kind offered by buxom, blue-eyed blondes,
for example! Finding good therapists in this way can be a bit hit and
miss. Personal recommendation is by far the best bet, but if not, contact the appropriate professional body for a list of approved practi-
tioners. Your library should have their addresses, or contact the
Institute for Complementary Medicine (see Appendix A).

Again, your GP might be a useful source for addresses. They
should be able to refer you to a homoeopath, and may know of suitable exercise, relaxation, meditation or yoga classes. They should also
be able to give you sound advice on diet and vitamin therapy, or be
able to recommend suitable books on these subjects. Do ask.

What to Ask the Therapist

After deciding which therapy or therapies to try, and finding someone
to contact, there are still things for you to find out. You know what
your needs are. The remaining question is, can this therapist fulfil
them? The only way to find out is to ask. Be well prepared for the initial consultation. Have your questions ready with the aim of finding
out whether they are going to be able to provide what you need.

Here are some questions you might like to ask:

- Can s/he describe to you the type of treatment?
- What are his/her general aims for the treatment?
- How can this treatment help you with your panic attacks?
- What results would s/he expect to see?
- What can you expect to happen in each session?
- How long are the sessions?
- How often would s/he expect them to be; once a week/twice a
  month etc.?

- What is the expected/average duration of the course of treatment?
- What are the advantages of this therapy over others?
- What can you expect to feel?
- What costs are involved?
- Does s/he offer concessionary rates? (If this is important for you)
- Does s/he do home visits? (Again, if this is important for you)

You might be able to think of other questions to ask. Make sure you cover them all in the consultation. You might want to take a notebook with you to jot down their answers. It is easy to forget what they say, especially if you go to see a number of different people.

How to Decide On a Therapist

Listen carefully to what each therapist says and the answers he or she gives. There is no need to make your decision at the end of the consultation. Take time to think about it. If they ask for a decision, simply say that you would like some time to think and will contact them shortly. I'm tempted to say that if they try to pressurize you, they are unlikely to be a good therapist and your answer should be 'No', but use your own judgement.

Besides the answers they have given, decide whether you actually like the person. You need to feel comfortable enough to trust your mind or body with them. The quality of the relationship between you will affect the success of the therapy, so decide if you like their attitude/manner/sense of humour/the level of understanding they show, and whatever else is important for you to find in that person. If you feel uncomfortable with them, go to another therapist.

Assess whether you think their aims meet yours. An assertiveness trainer may have a business-focused approach which would not meet your needs, or you might be looking for exactly that, but be talking to someone who aims to help people with intimate relationships.

And then there are the practical considerations like cost and convenience. Eventually, after looking at all these different aspects, you will hopefully be able to decide on a therapy which can provide just that extra little help and support you might have been looking for.

Some Suggestions

This is by no means a comprehensive list of all therapies which might be useful, but is included to serve as a springboard for you to use in your own research.

Aromatherapy

This uses essential oils (essences) extracted from plants. Different essences have different characteristics and can be used to treat a wide range of symptoms. A therapist either applies them directly to your skin through massage, makes a solution to be taken orally, or makes preparations for inhalation.

They are particularly useful with stress-related conditions, and may be of use in helping you achieve a state of calm. Bergamot, lavender, melissa, sandalwood and ylang-ylang are just some of the oils which are used to help relieve nervous tension.

Bach Flower Remedies

These are a type of medical herbal remedy and are available through some health food shops along with a free leaflet explaining what each is suitable for and what dosage to take. Examples are rock rose for alarm and panic; mimulus for fearfulness; white chestnut for obsessional thoughts or mental arguments. Rescue Remedy is a special formulation of five of the remedies and is useful in emergency-type situations. Karen used this and said that she found it 'successful' in helping with her panic attacks.

The remedies are aimed at treating emotional problems and are very safe to use; safe enough for self-medication. Despite this, you may prefer to see a therapist who can more accurately identify the correct prescription.

Biochemics

Within our tissues we have a number of inorganic salts. According to biochemic theory, we become ill when they are not in balance. Specific combinations of salts have been devised and are widely available through health food shops. Combination B may be of help to you: it is designed to alleviate edginess.

Tissue salts are safe to use in self-medication, and many homoeopaths use them.

Biofeedback

This has already been mentioned at various points throughout the book. Briefly, through self-monitoring your body's changes (e.g. heart rate, temperature) you can learn how to gain control over them. It teaches you how your mind-power can be used to bring about changes which previously you may have thought of as automatic. It may be particularly useful to people who panic, especially in learning how to take control over those distressing bodily symptoms which lead to attacks.

Biofeedback has been used with many ailments, but is particularly good with treating stress-related illnesses and may be of use to you.

Colour Therapy

Colour is around us all the time, and we subconsciously use it to affect or reflect our moods. Colour therapy seeks to use it for beneficial and remedial purposes, and may include eating appropriately-coloured food, drinking colour-energized water, colour breathing or coloured light bathing. A therapist can advise you on which colours to avoid and which to include in your life as simple aids to help minimize the risk of attacks.

Herbal Medicine

Herbs provide the historical basis for today's medical drugs. Using various parts of plants, a medical herbalist will make preparations in liquid, pill or ointment form to treat a wide variety of illnesses.

There may be a number of suitable herbal medicines to help relieve anxiety and stress. For example, valerian has a known tranquillizing effect.

Homoeopathy

A homoeopath treats the whole person. Although two people might have the same symptoms, they may be given different remedies. The pills, containing minuscule amounts of naturally-occurring substances, work on the principle of 'like treats like' – the symptoms each remedy is used to treat are the ones that a larger dose of this substance would cause in a healthy person.

Because of the infinitely small amounts of active constituents in the medication, they are completely safe to take and although some are available through chemists and health food shops, a professional consultation, diagnosis and prescription plan is better.

There are several preparations suitable for helping with panic attacks which a homoeopath might prescribe, such as arnica, opium or aconite, but appropriate medication really does depend on each individual.

Hypnosis

This is a means of inducing a trance-like state of suggestibility in a person. The altered state of mind allows post-hypnotic suggestions to be planted which, on waking, are carried out 'automatically', on cue. During hypnosis you are not necessarily unconscious, but remain fully aware of what the hypnotist is saying and doing.

Hypnosis is safe in the hands of a qualified practitioner, and may be of help with panic attacks, especially in learning how to cope in phobic situations. One woman I read about in my local paper who experienced panic attacks was so thrilled at the results she obtained from hypnotherapy that she wrote in to let others know about it.

Megavitamin Therapy

Vitamins are essential for our bodies to work efficiently and in harmony. We have already mentioned the importance of diet, since healthy eating helps us cope with the many stresses and strains in our daily lives.

Megavitamin therapy is used to treat a wide range of illnesses, carefully balancing the complex interaction of each vitamin with appropriate (but very high) doses. Evidence for megavitamin therapy is still sketchy, but may be of interest to you if you think your diet is severely lacking, especially in the vital B vitamins which help our nervous systems work efficiently. Self-medication with very high doses of vitamins is not recommended.

Neuro-Linguistic Programming (NLP)

This is a cognitive (thought) therapy which is aimed at empowering the individual to take control of their thoughts and actions and therefore their lives. It looks at self-defeating thought patterns and helps you replace them with more appropriate ones. Unlike traditional psychotherapies, it is fast acting.

It is useful in modifying behaviour patterns and may be of help if you want to learn about how to cope with phobic situations. It may also be of interest to you if you would like to investigate further the power of your mind, and learn how to use your thoughts more positively and productively in dealing with your panic attacks (and other aspects of your life).

Shiatsu (Acupressure)

Shiatsu is the finger massage of lines of energy which run throughout your body. A practitioner may massage just one specific acupuncture point or area, or may massage the whole body to realign and harmonize the flow of energy throughout.

The massage is gentle and, depending on your needs, can be either stimulating or sedating. It can be of use to people who panic, not only in calming and releasing bodily tension, but also through the practitioner's guidance on nutrition and open advice on improving your lifestyle.

Yoga

Exercise is important to keep your body working in harmony. Whatever happens to your body affects your mind, and vice versa. Yoga involves gentle movements aimed at making your body more supple and toned. It can also include mental 'exercises' aimed at learning self-control, similar in principle to biofeedback techniques. Respiration control is another aspect.

Yoga may be especially useful for panic attacks in all three areas: improving physical and mental well-being, learning about control, improving or correcting breathing (remember hyperventilation can be a contributory factor to the start of a panic attack in some people). Check it out.

Summary

♦ Some complementary therapies may be useful tools to include in your panic prevention kit.

♦ Know what your needs are from a specific therapy beforehand, then assess whether you think the practitioner can meet them.

♦ There are many sources of help available. Your GP and librarian may be good places to start.

♦ Mind and body work together. There are therapies available to help with both.

Section 3

13

What to Do When You Have an Attack

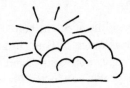

In the first two sections we brought panic attacks into the open and took a long look at them: what they are like, what might cause them, possible solutions, and the important role you have to play in them. In this final section I will discuss what you can do when you actually have one. I say 'when', because it would be foolish to pretend you won't. It would be leading you back into denial, which you may have employed as your only tactic until now. It's a negative perspective, and one which simply creates resistance and fear. Instead, accept that you may well have another attack.

This may appear to be a pessimistic statement if you haven't followed the book up to now, but I hope that those who have will appreciate the full meaning behind it. But let's just refresh our memories a little at this point. The key points to remember, which are going to be of use to you in handling an attack are:

◆ No harm will come to you. This is a statement of fact.
◆ The bodily sensations you feel are largely the result of too much adrenalin being in your bloodstream.
◆ The panic attacks are yours and because they are, you have the ability to take complete control over them.
◆ Thoughts which may prompt an attack, or which distress you during an attack, can also be brought under your control because they too are yours.

◆ Knowing that no harm will come to you, accept that an attack may happen, and if it does, go willingly into it. This shrewd tactic cleverly disarms any creeping feelings of fear. If you're not scared of PAM (the panic attack monster) you can see it for the squeaky, harmless little thing it is.

To handle attacks successfully, it might help if you have the attitude of wanting to find out as much as you can about them; really put them under the microscope; interrogate them through and through. In that respect, each one really is an incredibly valuable learning experience. When you next have one, you can now be really inquisitive about it. I thought it might be useful research for this book if I experienced another panic attack, but of course since I started looking forward to one I haven't come anywhere close. Here I am, with arms wide open to welcome an attack, and nothing happens. This might be a useful attitude for you to adopt. Go willingly into each one, with note pad in hand if necessary, and question it like fury once it's there, because you know it won't last for long, and soon it will be all over and then you'll have to wait until you have the opportunity again. If you don't take this approach, but start to back off in fear, the panic attack monster knows it has you in its grasp, just like school bullies do. Symptoms will appear worse hurling sensations at you like grenades, with greater and greater intensity. But if you sit there willingly, you're no game for them. So go into the attacks, and adopt an enquiring attitude. It may help defuse their ammunition.

In finding out all you can about attacks and their symptoms, as suggested earlier in the book, you may now realize that a certain pattern is beginning to emerge; your personal triggers and cues are perhaps becoming easier to recognize. If the attacks tend to start when you have been, or are, rushing around in headless chicken mode, become aware of your movements and purposefully slow them down. Coming to a halt and then starting again at a more relaxed pace can help ward off an attack. If you feel awkward about stopping abruptly, find some excuse: pretend to check the heel of your shoe; stop outside a shop window and fantasize about wearing the outfit in the window (which could be amusing if it's a hardware shop); stop to check in your pocket for your train ticket, even though you know it's there. Then, after a second or two, you can more easily flow into a more measured pace.

Movement and Distraction

Conversely, you may have become aware that thoughts of an attack start when you are doing nothing more energetic than having another cup of coffee (bad news in itself; see chapter 5). If this is the case, move around if you can and find a distraction as soon as you begin to feel uncomfortable. If you're in a meeting, turn to a new page and begin to write a letter/account of the meeting so far/shopping list/anything which gets you moving, however slightly. Pass around the water jug, or ask for it. Offer to open the window, or close the curtains. If you're at a party, go in search of a 1942 claret/plate of oysters/interesting person. It might be a futile search for any of them, but at least it gets you moving and directs your attention away from yourself.

Without knowing why, during my panic attacks I found great relief in jumping up and down, or running furiously on the spot, pumping my legs like a racing cyclist sprinting at the gun. Being a non-exercise type of person I was rather bemused that I should want to do something which was so uncharacteristic, but it really did help relieve the symptoms. Now that I know they are simply due to an excess of adrenalin which has prepared me for potentially intense physical activity (fight or flight), it makes sense that I should let my body respond in a way that was appropriate for it. Sprinting around the block may have been equally helpful in burning off this excess action fuel – adrenalin. Brian also reported finding that physical activity was useful: 'At work, going for a walk round the building would help'. You might like to try doing something the same when you next have an attack, to see whether it has a beneficial effect on you.

Movement may not always be convenient, but distraction always is. Concentrate on some object to take attention away from bodily sensations you are starting to notice. A chink in the curtains or a piece of rubbish on the floor will do. Question yourself about it: 'I wonder who/what/why/how/when/where . . .' For example, 'I wonder who lives in that house I can see through the chink in the curtains and what is going on there right now?' 'I wonder what sort of a life-cycle that piece of rubbish on the floor has?' 'I wonder why the director decided on that actor for the lead part?' 'I wonder where s/he bought that hat from?' 'I wonder how s/he made that punch and what ingredients s/he put in?' 'I wonder where that bus goes after my stop and what it looks like there?' Then try to give yourself answers; the more outrageous, the better. Put that incredibly fertile imagination of yours to good use and give it full rein. It might even lead you into some interesting ideas for writing a story, play or poem, making a film or painting a picture. Who knows? The important thing is to distract your attention and use up that mental energy in an alternative way, instead of directing it at yourself. Brian found an ingenious way of distracting himself from what he was experiencing by 'concerning myself with someone else's problems.' Similarly, Theresa finds that 'talking with people generally helps, as I am concentrating on something else.'

Another suggestion is to take advantage of the availability and social acceptability of personal stereos. Wearing one while walking around the supermarket, listening to your favourite, preferably calming, music may be a way of providing yourself with a pleasant distraction. You could also play back a recording of your own positive self-statements and affirmations. Commercially available relaxation tapes may be of some use, too. Try it out. It may or may not work, but you will come to no harm in trying, and if it does help you cope with difficult situations it could be just what you needed to break that cycle of panic attacks.

Hyperventilating

Hyperventilating has been associated with panic attacks. We have already looked at this, but it is worth returning to the subject. Whether hyperventilating causes panic attacks or whether it is one of the symptoms is to some extent academic. What is important is that learning how to control your breathing can help ameliorate the other symptoms, thereby reducing the full impact of the attack, especially when combined with other techniques in your repertoire such as acceptance and positive thought control. Jim found 'shifting your awareness to your breathing pattern' a good tactic to employ and Sandra used 'slow breathing during periods of intense unease'.

Turn to page 109 for a description of correct breathing and how to change yours. Once you become used to breathing using your diaphragm, you will find it quite easy to correct yourself when you notice feelings of unease prior to an attack. Even if you don't manage to correct it in time to ward it off, you can still use it as an effective way to minimize the impact of the attack itself.

Hyperventilating reduces the level of carbon dioxide in your blood. When this happens, it becomes part of the mechanism which triggers other panic symptoms. Therefore, some doctors suggest that increasing blood carbon dioxide levels may help. They recommend placing a paper bag (not plastic, please) over your nose and mouth, and breathing slowly and calmly, but not deeply, into it. We breathe out carbon dioxide, so taking back in what we have just exhaled into the bag is meant to redress the imbalance. Continue doing it until symptoms subside. I haven't tried this method myself, but Jenny found it very helpful and it was the treatment recommended by her doctor; along with moderate psychotherapeutic help. She learned how to recognize how she was hyperventilating, and so a paper bag became part of her panic attack tool kit. Try for yourself. It might be the missing item in yours.

Body and Mind

Chapter 10 stressed the importance of knowing your body's feelings. Prior to an attack this is important, because if you are aware of an uncomfortable tension in your muscles you can do something about it, before it has time to contribute to an escalation up the panic attack spiral. Hopefully, you will have taken the initiative and started to learn some relaxation techniques for inclusion in your prevention kit, perhaps through yoga classes. There are also commercially available tapes which talk you through relaxation exercises. They may be worth investigating. And when you have learned the techniques, you can call them into play to help you control muscle tension which can easily build up throughout the day, or in stressful situations.

As you are now aware, your mind's thoughts are also an important factor in the precipitation of an attack. It is worth stressing again that any thoughts you have are a) yours and yours alone, to do with as you will, and b) they are incredibly potent. To repeat chapter 8's chorus: a thought is a thing. Re-read that chapter if you feel you could do with some more reinforcement on that point. It is important for you to realize that the thoughts you may have, which keep you on a knife's edge of awareness and which help precipitate each attack, are yours. They do not happen of their own accord, although that is how we tend to think of them, as though they are separate entities over which we have no control. We do have control. You can make them do what you wish. Thoughts are your own internal voice, and you can make it say what you want in the same way you make your audible voice say either 'Good morning!' or 'What a beautiful day!'

Realizing this power you have over them gives you another immensely valuable tool for you to wield. We have already mentioned the positive effect of affirmations which can be used throughout the day, but the mind can also be used to channel supportive thoughts during, or just prior to, an attack.

When you first start to feel uncomfortable is the time when you may be tempted into allowing your thoughts to say 'This is the start of a panic attack. Here we go', or some such thing. I know that this has already been said in chapter 5, but it's worth stressing: do realize that those statements are your cue. It's like pressing the button on a gaming machine. As soon as you do, the tumble and jumble of sensations start and go wheeling out of control (or so it seems). Avoid pressing the button in the first place and you can save yourself a lot of bother. And you do that by having an alternative set of thoughts to replace the unhelpful ones which only serve to cue you into each attack.

At the point when you notice the initial symptoms (and this is where knowing your body self is important: what sensations alert you first?) you have the opportunity to reattribute them. What this means is that instead of thinking that your heavily beating heart means a panic attack, you could think one of these:

'I notice my heart's beating fast. It's not surprising, since I've been dashing around since midday.'

'I can feel my heart thumping. It's really interesting to see how it's reacting to those three cups of coffee I just drank.'

'My heart's racing a bit. How fascinating. It's true about alcohol. I understand now that four pints of beer really is a lot to drink on an empty stomach.'

'Here goes my heart; racing again. It's because I feel so excited about seeing this play. I've been looking forward to it for ages.'

I've used the example of heartbeats, but it may be that the first thing you tend to notice is heavy perspiration or feeling faint. The same thing applies. Tell yourself the real reason why you feel the way you do. For example:

'I've suddenly gone all sticky. Alcohol always makes me feel hot like this.'

'I feel so light-headed. Well, look. There aren't any windows open. No wonder.'

'I feel quite faint. But it's only because I skipped breakfast this morning.'

If you can't quite place the reason for why you might be feeling the sensations, remember about the important role adrenalin has to play. Reattributing your bodily sensations to it is also useful (and the truth). So, for example these might be statements you could use:

'I'm shaking all over, but now I know it's because of adrenalin.'

'My hands are tingling and I feel really peculiar. I've obviously got too much adrenalin in my system just now.'

'I feel so edgy. It must be an adrenalin excess again.'

Using these statements will prevent you from giving yourself the mental cue to start being scared at the prospect of another panic attack. Letting yourself know the reason for sensations you begin to experience will reassure you. Unlike the normal cues you use, these do not provide a reason to be fearful. How could you feel scared by simply confirming the real reason why your body is reacting in the way it is? You don't have to hope or believe that is the case. Know that it is true, and feel even more at ease in that knowledge.

Reinforce these thoughts by integrating some of the other things mentioned above. Relax your muscles, correct your breathing and then distract your thoughts away completely in the ways suggested.

This may be enough to avert a full attack, even though you may experience those initial physical sensations. However, there will be times, especially at first, when the attack may go into full swing until you get the hang of those pre-panic handling tactics. Don't despair at the prospect; there's no need to at all now, because of the things you have discovered. Recalling them during an attack, or certainly as you go into it, will help.

One of the most important things to remember is that you will come to no harm. Constantly tell yourself this. Attacks are unpleasant, but despite this, you know they really are all bark and no bite. And if you recall, what you are experiencing is the result of a protective measure your body has taken. The adrenalin it has released is in readiness to fight off any threats to you, or to take flight away from them. It is trying to keep you safe from harm. So how could you come to harm because of it? Remind yourself of this. You are not having a heart attack, you are not losing your mind, you are not about to lose control or faint. You might shake a bit, perspire heavily and have a strong heartbeat, but they can't harm you. There is nothing to be afraid of.

As you recall these things, take reassurance from them and stop trying to fight off these brave attempts your body is making to keep you safe. Accept what it is trying to do, and go with it instead. Even though your knees do feel wobbly, you know that it will eventually pass because it always does. If you can, try to take the opportunity to discover as much as you can about the attack while it is there. Be inquisitive about it; it will help you go into it. It will also provide you with more important 'inside' information which will be useful to you afterwards in helping you to understand it fully.

Chapter 7 was about the personal power you have over your self and your life. As you come to understand and accept this fully, it will help you with your attacks. They are within your control, because they are yours. You may not be able to control someone else's panic attacks, but yours belong to you and you can do with them what you will. Being fearful of them is a negative stance. Pro-actively deciding to accept them instead is a positive way forward, and evidence of you taking and exercising your control. It is a subtle shift in awareness, but is a vitally important one. Try to remember, and take reassurance from the fact that they are ultimately within your control; not by attempting to repress them, but by acceptance of both them and your own personal power.

Use your positive affirmations to help remind you of these things. Be your own friend and support. Learn to trust in yourself – you will be much more reliable than a pill or sip of water or alcohol. And the pay-offs are much better.

You may now want to read this chapter again. You know what you are like before and during an attack, so it is up to you now to develop your safety net plan of action. A number of options are suggested here which may be of help to you. Work out which ones you think will be of help to you in particular, and which you feel you could easily use. If you know your mind seems to become particularly confused during an attack, then giving yourself just one or two positive things to recall will be enough for you to begin with. If you feel that you would particularly appreciate doing something physical, then you can look forward to trying those suggestions out next time and think about integrating the mental exercises later.

I have already mentioned the importance of you being fully aware of your self and your lifestyle. Use that knowledge now to prepare your plan. For example, if you know that one or two situations only tend to precipitate an attack, develop positive plans of action tailored to suit them and what you do there. Start to make those plans now and notice how you can already sense a feeling of getting in touch with your personal power. Begin to feel that you are taking control. This is you being pro-active. This is you moving forward.

Summary

♦ Trying to fight against a panic attack is negative. Take proactive action instead to make positive moves forward.

♦ Accept that you will have another attack, and start to develop your own carefully-thought-out plan of action and way of dealing with it.

♦ There are no 'failed' attempts – there are only opportunities to experience and to learn.

14

If You're on Your Own

We have now looked at what you can do to deal successfully with future panic attacks. The suggestions apply to everyone, and you can choose from them which ones are most suitable for you. Quite rightly it has focused on you, your bodily sensations and your thoughts, but we also need to consider the personal circumstances surrounding each situation in which you have one. This chapter will look at the issues involved in having an attack when you are on your own, and chapter 15 will look at your attacks in relation to your friends and family.

The fear of having an attack when you are on your own is one which hasn't been mentioned yet. From my own experience, I know this can be a potent one. It layers itself on top of the other fears you may already have about the actual attack itself. For me it seemed to paint a picture of the worst scenario I could imagine (there was my fertile imagination being put to no good again!) I remember one attack I had when I was travelling to Greece to join some friends who had gone there on holiday the week before. Unfortunately, work had prevented me from going at the same time, but I knew I needed a good break so although I had never travelled abroad on my own before, the prospect of eventually sitting on a sun-drenched beach, miles away from the source of my worries but only yards away from a taverna, inspired me on.

Obviously I hadn't acknowledged how excited but also how anxious I was about doing the trip, which involved a train, a plane, a connection to a ferry, and a ferry trip out to an island somewhere, and then an attempt to find the hotel. I was anticipating the language barrier to be a problem. Would I be able to recognize the sign for Naxos written in the Greek alphabet, I wondered, or would I end up on Paros, Milos or Karos?

Feelings of unease started on the train to the airport. Trying to fight down the sensations, I eventually came unstuck when I got off the train and reached the glaring lights inside the airport where the thought came rushing through, swifter than the train I'd just been on, that I would be on my own on the plane and for the rest of the journey until I (hopefully) reached my destination. This thought of being alone provided the final cue for which my attack was looking, and off it went.

The thought of being on your own can be additional fuel to stoke up background anxieties. You start to anticipate situations where you might be on your own and therefore equate them with having an attack. This specific fear can then work on two levels: as an immediate thought cue, and as a 'what if' worry to fuel anxiety prior to the next attack.

Tracking my thoughts back to that time, I know that it seemed less fearful to think of having an attack when I knew someone was to hand. You might feel the same. For example, Theresa, a young, single, assistant lawyer living on her own acknowledges that 'having no-one around became part of the problem'. And someone like Jimmy, 15 years old and still at school at the time, found that being on his own was the only time when he had panic attacks. Perhaps your experience of how awful the attacks are makes you want to have someone there to support you through them. Previously, without knowing what the attacks were and believing you were going to die or have a heart attack, you could be forgiven for not wanting to be alone. Let's face it, who would want to think of dying with no one around? Who would phone for the ambulance? Would you end up writhing on the floor for hours or days in agony before your last breath came? I never voiced the thoughts in so many words, but that is what fleetingly passed through my mind and manifested itself as a fear of having an attack on my own.

This whole issue brings to mind one of the theories of causation mentioned in chapter 4, linking panic attacks to separation anxiety. This may begin in childhood and be the result of having to face demanding situations without the supportive presence of a parent or some other significant person. The similarity between this and the fear of having to face a panic attack without the support of another person seems quite clear. The theory is supported by the fact that some people experience their first attacks after the real or threatened loss of an important relationship.

This may explain why the thought of having a panic attack when you are on your own can fill you with even more fear and anxiety. It might be rekindling this basic unresolved dread of facing a demanding situation without the strong support of someone else being there. There are two things which might help to counter this particular fear. One is to accept that anyone who has a panic attack has it on their own. They can't share it with others. So even if, for example, you have an attack while sitting at the dinner table, you will still be experiencing it on your own, regardless of who or how many people you might be with. Others might not even notice you're having one. What I am trying to stress is that there is nothing special about being on your own and having a panic attack. The attack will still just run its course and eventually subside. It will not be any worse because you are on your own, although your fear beforehand might cue one to start. Otherwise, the attack will be experienced in the same way as if you were with friends/family/a room full of close colleagues.

The other fear which I had was the thought about the practicalities which I mentioned above. Who would phone for the doctor/ ambulance/undertaker? This was before I understood what the attacks were and what had caused them. In my fear through ignorance, my vivid imagination thought the worst. Because like you, I now understand the reasons why, and that the attack will not harm me, I could rationalize that thought if I had it again. Back to reattribution, and back to 'a thought is a thing'. Now you know you will be all right, that it will pass without doing you any lasting damage, you can forget about thinking you need someone there to rescue you from death's door. You won't need anyone because you're not going to be at death's door, and never will be because of a panic attack.

Think over these things and perhaps read through them again until you really do understand, know and accept these facts. They are powerful tools for your panic prevention kit.

Living on Your Own

Until you have fully accepted those facts, the prospect or the reality of living on your own may seem a rather less than attractive proposition than it would otherwise. However, it is an excellent, positive position to be in. Not convinced?

Living on your own offers so many more opportunities for you to tackle panic attacks than if you were living with other people, either friends or family. Indeed, other people may be the cause of some problem areas and create anxiety in those who live with them. Think back to what was said in chapter 9, for example, about those who like to undermine confidence in others.

Chapter 11 stressed the importance of your lifestyle and the impact it can have on panic attacks. Hopefully, after reading that chapter you have begun to look closely at those elements in the way you live your life which might be working against you being free from attacks. It is too easy, as I know, to fall into unhealthy and unhelpful habits when you only have yourself to account for. Indulgence shows its negative face.

Giving yourself only good things which please you reinforces your self-worth positively. For example, ordering what you want to eat from the menu, even if it is the most expensive item, is saying that you are worth it. Ordering the cheapest (not because of lack of money or because you want that particular dish) is the same as saying you are not. Reinforcing your self-worth is important, but indulging in things which only serve to expand your waistline, or make you drunk, or deny your body the vitamins and minerals it needs to stay healthy, is not something which shows you value yourself. You might like to pause here and think about those things which are excessive in your life and which negate your self-worth.

Your feelings of self-worth start in childhood. What responsibilities do parents believe they have to their children? To love them and keep them warm, safe and secure may be top of the agenda; to provide opportunities for them which they as children might have missed out on, for whatever reason; to develop a clone image of themselves and successfully transfer their values onto them. These may or may not be worthy aims. But one thing that is important is whether parents assume the responsibility of helping their children become fully-functioning independent human beings, who know how to make their own decisions and how to cope effectively with mistakes. I wonder how many parents actively encourage independent thought and how many make sure their children have the life skills necessary for them to pass successfully and happily through into adulthood? It is during childhood that learning about the practicalities of life and about how to value your self-worth should take place. Perhaps you feel it didn't happen to you.

But we are dynamic beings, never static and always able to change and adapt. If you think you may not have been given appropriate instruction in life skills which should be your self-protection and self-support through life, you might like to start changing now and begin to strengthen those areas in which you feel weak or lacking. Start to make those lifestyle changes which will lead to a more supportive and pleasurable environment for yourself.

The point I want to make is that those people who are sharing their lives with others might find it far more difficult to make those necessary and perhaps major lifestyle changes. Instead of being free to modify their eating/sleeping/social habits literally overnight, they may have to negotiate through possibly conflicting demands and needs from others. If you live on your own you are unfettered by such restrictions. You are in an ideal position to make as many positive changes as you like in as short a space of time as you want. And change them back again. Or try something completely different next week. The choice is yours.

Chapter 9 looked at the importance of self-confidence in dealing with panic attacks. Unfortunately, partners and friends are not necessarily always helpful in massaging others' self-confidence, and some positively seek to undermine it. It is important to recognize this, and understand that people who are like that have problems of their own. For whatever reason, there are those who like to pull others down, attempt to deflate their enthusiasm, ridicule their successes, find fault with what you do, or give insincere praise. These people are too negative to do your self-confidence any good. Another exercise in taking control of your life and giving yourself more self-worth is to decide not to accept their comments. This may mean excluding those people from your life altogether, or alternatively, learning assertiveness skills so that you can rebuff or challenge them. In the meantime it might be worth keeping in mind what Eleanor Roosevelt said, that 'no one can make you feel inferior without your consent'.

Dealing with relationships which undermine rather than support is more difficult if you live with the person or people concerned. Years of such abuse may have built up, and will take some time to change and modify. It may be more difficult in such circumstances to outwardly become a challenging new you. When you live on your own it is much easier to identify those things you want to change – and then to go about doing it. It is easier when you live on your own to decide which friends and colleagues are supportive, and to concentrate on them while relegating the unsupportive ones to a more suitable position. You can develop plans of action and try them out without the threat of someone's unkind words to knock your confidence back on the ground again. You have the freedom to explore, try out new things and begin to develop at last, with only yourself to please. You are in a very fortunate position.

What ultimately develops from this is a sense of how much personal power you actually have. In this environment you have the freedom to start spreading those wings which may have been clipped by unkind or unsupportive parents or which you were never taught how to use. Living on your own offers exciting circumstances in which to make those changes which you know may help you successfully learn how to deal with your panic attacks.

Other Lifestyle Changes

Besides the suggestions in the chapter on lifestyle, there are others which may be useful for you to consider if you live on your own.

In terms of helping to reduce anxiety levels, you could consider getting a cat or dog. Studies have shown the beneficial effect having a pet can have on people. I know myself that it is certainly very soothing and comforting to have my cat climb up, nuzzle against my cheek, curl round and fall asleep, purring, in my lap as I stroke her and give her a good scratch behind the ears. You might like to think about whether a pet might be something for you to consider. They don't suit everyone, and dogs especially need a lot more exercising and looking after than cats do. But it might be effective in distracting your attention away from yourself and helping reduce your anxiety levels.

When asked for suggestions which he might give to others who have panic attacks and who live on their own, Jimmy quite simply answered 'consider living with others'. I would agree with this, but with a proviso. Just as the negative way of dealing with an attack is to escape from or avoid the situation, so deciding to look for someone to live with could be for negative reasons. Think it through. Do you really want to lose all those opportunities which have just been outlined and which could positively help you with your panic attacks? Would sharing your life make more problems than it would solve? Would you expect sharing to cure your panic attacks? Be aware of what sharing might mean. However, if you decide from a position of strength and sure inner knowledge that you are positively happy to share with others and that is what you really want in life, then why deny yourself that enjoyment? So long as you don't expect it to be 'The Answer'.

Theresa suggested 'keep active; have friends around, go out and do things. Try not to feel sorry for yourself by sitting alone pondering on it,' while Brian suggested 'visit friends often. Find an absorbing hobby,' and then added 'don't sit indoors worrying'. It is important for everyone to develop outside interests. Think about whether you could happily incorporate some new activities into your life. It might be something which takes you outside your home, or you might prefer a home-based hobby, like Brian suggested. When you are totally absorbed in an activity you enjoy, you can experience an altered state of consciousness, similar to what happens during meditation. Meditating reduces anxiety. Sitting on the floor in a lotus position isn't the only way to do it.

However, developing interests outside the home has additional benefits. You are more likely to widen your experiences and expand your range of social contacts. It may be worth your while considering what you could take up, and the very positive effect it might have on your life. A trip to your local library should enable you to find out about local classes, clubs and activities you could join. Pay them a visit. A browse among their bookshelves could also give you some ideas for a new hobby or interest to take up.

Being without a partner may be something which you have identified as making you unhappy and which you want to change. I would be tempted to say the same things about this as I did about deciding to share living accommodation with people. If it is done from a positive stance, fine. If, however, you want a partner in order to save you from your panic attacks and to provide 'The Answer' in the same way you might hope living with friends might do, then you could be in for a let-down. But if you know you want a partner because you prefer to positively share your life, then do something about it. Many people will simply bemoan the lack of a special person in their life without doing much about it. If you really do want to meet someone then be pro-active. Realize that if you are not meeting people in the way you live your life now, then you need to start doing things which will allow you to. And if you have your sights set on marriage, do consider joining a dating agency. Many people do, so why can't you?

You might have to work harder at making your social life work when you live on your own, but you are at least in a better position to choose those things which you really enjoy doing, and which make you feel good about yourself and your life. When you begin to feel good about things, your anxiety levels drop and when that happens you instantly reduce the risk of another panic attack. Start to think about other things you could start to include in your life which would make you feel good.

During an Attack

The beginning of this chapter talked about the needlessness of fearing an attack on your own. Hopefully this will have reassured you. Having an attack is the same for everyone, regardless of who you may or may not be with, so the suggestions in the previous chapter about what to do during one should be of equal help to you, too.

As you begin to develop your own successful ways of averting and dealing with attacks, your fear will begin to recede. But until that time, you may want to have some additional support. Having identified those friends, relatives and colleagues with whom you feel confident, you are now in a position to ask them for some direct support if you haven't done so already. True friends are only too willing to help in times of distress. Talk to them about your attacks and ask them if you could call on them if you ever need to. Just knowing they would be there at the end of a phone if you wanted to call might be enough to allay some of your fears. I occasionally used to telephone my sister during an attack. I could barely speak, so I just asked her to talk away for a few minutes. Hearing her voice while she went on about what she'd had for dinner and what work had been like brought a sense of calm and 'normality' to me. The familiarity of it all seemed to ground me again. There is more about the role of relatives and friends in the next chapter, but certainly if you think this would help you go through your next attack then do it. Use the opportunity of that support to really go in to the attack, to accept and flow with it. Whoever is acting as your support will not be the answer to your attacks, and you have to be careful not to think of their help in that way. But they can be a support to you while you learn how to handle your attacks more positively.

If it is inconvenient for you to phone during an attack, you could ask someone to do a tape recording for you, either reading aloud a relaxation exercise or just speaking reassuring words to you. You can then play it back during an attack. You could also try recording your own affirmations, spoken in a firm, positive voice and saying those things which you know would be helpful to hear when you're going through one. Also, physical reassurance might be important to you. If so, you could try squeezing a cushion or pillow. It's not quite the same as having a hand to hold, but it is soft and comforting and it might help. Try it. If it does help, combine it with your selection from the other suggestions which now form part of your personalized tool kit.

Summary

- At the end of the day, all of us are alone in handling our panic attacks, even if we are with other people.
- Take comfort from knowing that all of us are alone, not just you, and therefore paradoxically we are all together.
- Since you now understand the attacks better and know no harm will come to you, there is nothing special to fear about having an attack on your own.
- There are lots of benefits to living on your own in learning about your panic attacks and how to handle them. It's up to you to see the opportunities it presents and to use them.
- It is all right to ask for support from friends and relatives. Good ones will give it willingly.

15

For Friends and Relatives

This chapter is primarily for your friends and relatives. They can be an enormous help and support – or a hindrance. Without a supportive network one can feel vulnerable at the best of times, so while you learn how to deal with your panic attacks, knowing you have helpful people around will be a great asset. Studies show that good support from those we are closest to really does help reduce stress and indirectly improves health. So for you they may be doubly useful. However, they need to know what to do, which is why the chapter is written for them.

Making It Easier For Those You Know

If you find your partner or friends are unwilling to take the time to become too involved in the whys and wherefores, yet appear to be sympathetic and express a willingness to be of help, you may have to take the initiative. Spend five minutes, or however long it takes, to explain to them what you now know about what the attacks are, to help them understand the basics. You could just say that they happen when you have too much adrenalin in your system, which makes you feel nervy and uncomfortable. Then tell them what you would like them to do next time, or perhaps between times. If you experience feelings of insecurity or lack of confidence in certain situations, you could ask them for their support to help you build your confidence. People like to know what is expected of them, and you explaining what you want will make it easier.

The rest of the chapter is addressed to your friends and/or relatives. Let them read it.

The Impact the Attacks Have On You

Being nearest and dearest to someone who has panic attacks must be very difficult. You may have noticed over time that he or she has changed because of the attacks, leaving you bewildered and confused. They may have modified their life quite drastically to accommodate the attacks, and you may have felt the impact of that on yourself. It is understandable that as the panic attacks have continued, with perhaps few signs of progress, the person you know has begun to withdraw into his- or herself, and even begun to appear to you to be quite self-centred. Their concern about how situations will affect them, how anxious they are feeling, what they can and can't do, can be difficult to accept. Although it may look like self-indulgence, it has, in the past, been their attempt at trying to cope and make life livable. Your reaction to this may have been to withdraw and 'let them get on with it'. You may also have become angry with them, faced with what you might interpret as 'not trying', sheer self-pity or even bloody-mindedness. With both of you previously being in the dark about the attacks, this is understandable. But for them, your attitude may have had the effect of making them feel guilty about the impact their attacks have on you. They may also have begun to feel weak, pathetic and ineffectual, even that they might be imagining the attacks. People who have panic attacks tend to accept blame only too easily.

It is important that you acknowledge and accept the negative feelings you have been having. Bearing in mind the lack of guidance and knowledge of what to do, which both of you have had to cope with, it is understandable that you should have felt frustrated; not only with your partner or friend, but also with yourself. Hopefully, this book will have started to give them some insight to help them move forward. Gradually you might begin to feel the impact of this positive change. It will provide you with the opportunity to take more positive action, which might help relieve your sense of anger and frustration at not knowing what to do for the best.

Perhaps the first thing to realize is that the panic attacks belong to the person who experiences them. Although you can play an important part in helping him or her to find ways to bring them to an end, you are not the person responsible for the attacks; they are. After reading this book through, they should be aware of this fact by now. Perhaps that makes you feel better already. Shrug off that responsibility; it isn't yours.

You may have felt that the panic attacks have come to exert a powerful control, not only over your friend or partner but also over your own life. This will undoubtedly have created feelings of resentment. With a new direction in sight, this should now begin to change. Indeed, it must. Panic attacks ought not to be allowed to control anyone, and as your partner begins to find their own sense of control this should gradually come to an end. Certainly it is important for you to continue to do things you want to do, and if they choose not to join in, it should not affect your decision.

Although the panic attacks don't belong to you, you are close to the person to whom they do belong, and exert a certain amount of influence. You may have a part to play in the attacks themselves. I'm certainly not saying they are your fault or responsibility: they can't be, because they're not yours. But it might be worthwhile taking an honest look at what the attacks mean to you. You may say that you would like to see them go, but in fact they may be serving a useful purpose, of which you are probably not consciously aware. They could be a barrier to other more serious issues which are being avoided. You might unconsciously like someone being dependent on you because of them. That position might make you feel good; it might make you feel wanted. You might even wonder whether you would still be wanted without the excuse of the panic attacks. And although it has been mentioned that panic attacks can exert a certain amount of control over people's lives, someone having them could provide a means for you to control them and their life, even though you may never have realized it.

These issues may not apply to you, but it is still worthwhile examining what role you play, what the panic attacks mean to you and whether they serve some other purpose. Carl and Stephanie Simonton, in their work with cancer patients, comment that the whole family often has a part to play in the onset of the disease – the family itself has cancer, but just one person ends up with the symptoms.

What You Can Do, In General

We can now look at helpful things to do when someone has a panic attack. But do bear in mind that we're talking here about an ideal way to help. Try the best you can but remember that no one expects perfection from you.

It is vitally important that you understand as much about panic attacks as your friend/partner/relative. Without knowledge, feelings of confusion and resentment about their behaviour might persist. It will be much easier for you to be supportive if you know more of what the attacks are about. So if you haven't done so already, do read the rest of this book. Afterwards, discuss it with them, and find out what strategies they are developing as a result of them reading it. Use supportive and encouraging words about their plan of action. It is theirs and it is important you show it respect. It may not be how you would do it, but you are not that person. They know what they want to do, and have chosen the most appropriate starting point for them. After reading the whole of this book you will appreciate the need for them to build their own sense of confidence which may be lacking. They need to learn how to spread their wings in order to find out how powerful they are, and how much power they have over their attacks. Your new role is to support them while they progress through this important phase, and respecting their choice of strategies is the start of this.

The rest of this book may also help you be prepared for, and appreciate, the changes which they may begin to make to their life.

You will be less resistant to or threatened by such changes if you understand why they are happening.

Reassure and confirm that you do want to help them in the work they will be doing on their panic attacks. Don't take it for granted that they will assume you want to, just because you have read about it. Tell them you're right behind them in what they do. Ask them what they would like you to do to help; not only during an attack, but also in terms of support at other times. Asking them will help develop their sense of responsibility about their attacks and a feeling of taking control over their situation.

It might be tempting, in trying to help, to want to do things for them. You care about this person, and it's a natural instinct to try to save someone from encountering anguish or difficulties. But remember that the attacks are not your responsibility, and neither is the learning process. You cannot do it for them. Your job is to encourage and support them in their own attempts and help them develop feelings of self-confidence and self-mastery. This can't happen if you do things for them all the time. It only encourages avoidance behaviour, which keeps them outside potential learning situations.

Encourage them to do things for themselves as much as possible. Haranguing them to attempt something which is obviously beyond their present capabilities will not help, but jollying them along into attempting something new will. It needn't be anything ambitious. They need to feel secure in their abilities to cope, so relatively undemanding situations might be best at first while they find their footing, and try out their new skills and strategies. Friends can help by continuing to invite them along to join in with activities. Knowing that friends are there, ready for when they feel up to it, may help provide a goal for which to aim. Accept that they will probably continue to turn down the invitations or excuse themselves at the last minute, but that is fine. That is their choice and you must respect it. They will come along in their own good time when they know they are ready for it. But it will only add to their levels of anxiety if they are made to feel guilty for saying 'No, thank you' or 'Sorry, I've changed my mind.'

Acknowledge all their attempts in the way you feel would be most appropriate. It will help a great deal. You can encourage progress by countering negative statements and attitudes which they might make, perhaps in despair at an apparent 'failure' or the slow progress being made. Remind them at regular intervals of how far they have come and the real progress they have made so far. You might like to re-read about affirmations in chapter 8. You could develop some of your own which you could use to counter negativity. For example, 'You are still in control', 'You are getting better and better', 'You are strong and capable', and even a simple 'I love you'. Try to work out some of your own.

Learning how to relax is an important part of reducing anxiety levels. You might like to join in with them to learn and do the exercises together. Are there any other things you can do to help create a relaxing environment for them? People learn by example. Think about how much positive relaxation you have in your own life. Perhaps you could do with some more, too. Develop your own strategies for relaxing more, and draw their attention to what you are doing and how good it is making you feel. It could provide them with the ideas or confidence to do the same, or something similar but which is more in keeping with their own personal preferences.

Learning how to give a massage could be useful, and something which you could enjoy together. Touch is a potent way of reducing stress and anxiety. Even a simple hug, a squeeze of the arm, or holding someone's hand helps. Holding and rocking the person, if they are feeling particularly vulnerable, is incredibly comforting. However, having said that, some people are uncomfortable with what they see as excessive spontaneous shows of physicality. You must use your own judgement, based on how well you know them. Ask them if that is what they like.

Massage is not only pleasurable but it also positively helps you unwind, relax and ease away the tension you might not even know you had. People who panic tend to have high levels of anxiety, and giving them a massage could help a lot in reducing those levels. Giving you a massage may have the advantage for them of helping to detract from their own worries and concerns. There are lots of useful books available to show you how. Visit your local library. Or you could find a local class to go to. For relaxing massage, the techniques are simple and easy to pick up and could be an investment for both of you.

Touching can also be a way of opening doors to more successful verbal communication. Encourage them to talk about their fears, worries and concerns. Jenny clearly identifies this as a great help to her: 'As time went on I learned to talk about a problem before it got to be a *worry* [her emphasis]. When I shared my worry with my husband it always seemed so much smaller afterwards . . . more often than not it [a panic attack] was through me worrying or being upset about something.' Through learning to communicate her worries and share them, Jenny made great progress with her attacks. You could help the person you know in the same way. 'But I have enough worries of my own,' you might moan. The aim of listening to someone else's fears and concerns is not to provide the answers (they have them within, anyway). Nor is it to weep and wail alongside. If you have ever been severely upset over something yourself, then you will realize doing that isn't particularly helpful. No, the aim is simply to listen and encourage them to talk openly and express their feelings. It isn't for you to judge or decide for them what they should do – that's their responsibility. Yours is to simply be there while they 'get things off their chest'. You are a sounding board – and perhaps a provider of tissues. This is what psychotherapists do. They don't provide any answers, but they do give a secure environment in which to voice worries and troublesome thoughts, and through careful questioning encourage a fuller investigation and expression of feelings.

Many people are brought up to think that openly expressing emotions is somehow wrong or bad. Like water, dammed emotions will attempt to find a chink through which to flow freely. If they can't, they can raise anxiety to danger levels. You can help by encouraging your partner to express their emotions and by reassuring them that it is all right to do so. If you really feel inadequate to cope with this, you could encourage them to find a professional who could help. But at the very least, you could encourage positive emotions like laughter, which is incredibly therapeutic. I have already mentioned Norman Cousins, who remedied his illness not only through vitamin C but also through laughter. *Smile Therapy* by Liz Hodgkinson (Macdonald Optima, 1987) is an interesting read and could give you some ideas for ways of increasing your own levels of enjoyment, too. But the most important thing to aim for is to encourage communication and keep those lines open.

What to Do During an Attack

You may now realize that an attack can be prompted by anxious thoughts simply about the possibility of an attack. Worries about the situation in which it might happen can be strong enough for him or her to decide that they would rather avoid going there. You might be able to help at this stage, before they get into that situation and before an attack manifests itself.

The worries they have will be very real to them. Ignoring them may make the person feel isolated, and it could rekindle deep-seated fears linked to separation anxiety. Chapter 4 explains in more detail what this is. So instead of ignoring the worries, acknowledge them. Listen to what their fears are about, but make it clear that you are unwilling to let the fears control things. Reassure your partner/friend of your support and love but also let them see that you do not accept an escalation of worries. Be firm, and if necessary simply tell them to stop worrying. It is a difficult path to tread because you need to show you care, yet your aim is to discourage them from unnecessary fretting. Be firm, but be affectionate with it. And just try the best you can.

Reassure them by getting them to explain again what their strategies are to be in the event of an attack. It will help them feel prepared and take away some of the fear of not being able to cope, or of losing control. After they have explained, encourage them to realize that they will know what to do even if they do have one. You might like to suggest doing some relaxation exercises together beforehand, and remind them of their positive affirmations. Focus on the positive aspects of whatever situation it is they are worried about: the friends they might be meeting, the reviews of the film, and say how excited you feel, too. It may help them reattribute the fluttering sensations they have in their tummy when they hear you say that's how excitement makes you feel.

As much as you can, try to forget about the possibility of an attack. Nervously checking and watching them will only put them on edge and keep their focus on themselves. Even ignore the first signs of an attack and help divert their attention, either through encouraging a different train of thought or by visual distraction or by getting them to move around with a purpose; not 'to stop you having an attack' but perhaps because you've 'just noticed something really interesting over there' which you want to show them.

However, there will be times when an attack goes into full swing. Hopefully, you will have talked beforehand about what they prefer you to do during one. Jenny said she '. . . found it extremely comforting to get my husband to hold my hand and to talk to me.' Brian wanted shows of 'genuine concern' to reassure him. But Theresa thought that 'to have someone fussing over me won't help me to overcome it.' This was echoed by Colin who wanted 'nothing at all really. Just to leave me on my own. To let me be on my own so I could fall asleep and try and relax the panic attack feeling away.' Myself, I wanted contact with someone. If I was alone I would telephone my sister or a good friend and get them to talk away to me while I simply listened. Otherwise, I would hold hands or have someone hug me. It seems that we all know what we want others to do during an attack, but there is little consensus of what that might be. So it is important for you to know beforehand what your friend/partner finds most comforting and most helpful. Suddenly making physical contact with someone who prefers to sit quietly alone might only make matters worse!

Remind them of what their present strategies are: perhaps accepting it and going into it fully, or changing their breathing pattern. Also remind and reassure that they know no harm will come to them; they know it will pass; that they are handling it well; and any positive statements which you know are particularly apt for the person concerned. Reassurance is important in helping to take away the fear of what might be happening to them and although they should be reminding themselves of this, hearing someone else say the same may help reinforce the message.

After an Attack

You may be tempted to want to handle them like porcelain after the attack has subsided. Instead, continue with positive statements, that they have come through that one all right; that they stayed in control; that they are still in control; and get them back into the activity/situation if they had to leave. This last is important to remove the risk of avoidance behaviour setting in. It may be best not even to ask whether they want to return, but perhaps just take it for granted that you both will and while still talking, go back in. Forcing them and making an issue of it will be counter-productive, so be aware of the distinction. Then forget about it. Try not to tiptoe around as if another attack might happen. Your forgetting will help them to do the same.

Outside the situation, perhaps in the security of familiar surroundings, you could encourage them to talk about the experience. There is always something to be learned from each one, and if they appear to have forgotten that, do remind them. This time they may have delayed leaving the situation, or have been quicker at going back in. They may have remembered their positive self-statements or managed to distract themselves for longer. They might have realized this time that they came even nearer to really letting go or remembered that they meant to watch their thoughts and forgot, or that they had one cup of coffee too many. All this information is useful and gives a positive resolution of how well they have done and how they are better prepared for the next time. Your encouragement, support and positive attitude at this point will help enormously. But don't let them dwell on it and once the ground has been covered, move the conversation and activity on to something else.

Depending on how close you are to the person you know with panic attacks, you might feel strained yourself at times. It is important that you look after yourself well. You will be less than useless if you become ill through ignoring your own wants and needs. So make sure you do things you enjoy, and remember that the panic attacks are not in control of either you or your life.

It may help relieve any mental stress you might feel by also recalling that the panic attacks are not your responsibility, and neither is that person's life. We each are our own responsibility, and your friend or relative has more than adequate resources to make progress with their attacks. Chapter 7 reinforces that message. Instead, your role is simply to provide supportive words and encouraging gestures. The rest is up to them, but your positivity can help them realize it.

Summary

◆ Read the rest of the book.
◆ The panic attacks are not your responsibility.
◆ Acknowledge any difficult feelings you may have concerning their panic attacks. The reasons are understandable.
◆ Look at what the attacks may mean to you on a subconscious level.
◆ Understand what your role is and the most helpful things you can do.
◆ Try to be supportive but independent; loving but firm.

16

Children and Panic Attacks

I said in chapter 2 that panic attacks tend to be experienced by people between the ages of 15 and 40. In the younger age range, many people start to develop attacks around the age of 16, although for some they occur before then. One study revealed that children as young as four years old experienced them. We may tend to think of panic attacks as being an adult thing, but this obviously isn't the case.

The study just mentioned looked at nearly three hundred children and teenagers, between the ages of four and 19. They were all psychiatric patients who had been referred for different reasons such as problems with obsessions or anti-social behaviour – not for panic attacks. But the researchers discovered that 26 per cent of them, that is, over a quarter, experienced panic attacks. This doesn't mean that a quarter of all children have them, but it does confirm that youngsters do have attacks, and there is a likelihood that they may be linked to other problems.

There are some medical specialists who have queried whether children, especially very young ones, really do have panic attacks as such. However, although they may not feel fear before or during an attack as adults tend to, they can still experience the same bodily sensations as the rest of us. Lack of fear is perhaps not surprising. Children, in their innocence, often do things which adults wouldn't dare, simply because adults have a greater ability to anticipate danger and catastrophes. There must be many parents who have swept their child out of a potentially dangerous situation, followed by wails of confusion as their 'innocent' adventure (climbing out on the upstairs window-sill, for example) comes to a sudden end. So although children's perception of what they experience may not be labelled by them as panic, the description of what actually happens to them physically does fit.

Personality

Just as there are theories about a 'panic personality' in adults, there are similar ideas about children. It has been observed that they tend to be rather quiet, timid and nervous of speaking out. Like adults, they may feel a severe lack of confidence. They have a tendency to think very poorly of themselves, and that they are lacking in many areas. Ideas they have about themselves are negative and self-critical. For example, they might think they do very badly at school, whereas the truth is they are doing well. Expectations they have of themselves, and those they think others have of them, to excel and achieve are at the root of such self-critical feelings.

Because of their poor levels of self-confidence, they are particularly sensitive towards criticism and rejection, and may avoid doing anything which they think might incur it. If they don't think they will be able to do something successfully, then they won't even try, for fear of failing. So instead of being bold and daring, as most children are in the thrill and excitement of childhood with so much to explore and discover, they tend to hold back from taking risks.

Holding themselves back in this way because of their poor self-image, lack of self-confidence, fear of failure and all they think would come in its wake, they sow the seeds for developing very high levels of anxiety.

As you can see, there are many similarities between these observations of children who panic and traits which tend to appear in adults who have panic attacks.

Identifying Possible Panickers

As children develop and grow, learning more about themselves and their environment, it is only natural that occasionally they will have experiences which cause them worry. With loving care and support, the worries tend to be resolved pretty quickly, and are soon forgotten in the rush to discover the next excitement. But worries which become excessive can cause problems. Avoidant behaviour may develop as a result, and may be linked with experiences of panic attacks, much as it is with adults. School phobia is a commonly-observed avoidant behaviour in children. The links between this and panic have been suggested, based on adults with panic disorder frequently reporting having experienced school phobia in the past.

This, and other avoidant behaviour, may be warning signs to look out for.

What Makes Children Worry?

There are many situations which can easily provoke feelings of anxiety in children and, as is to be expected, the majority of their worries revolve around their immediate environment: personal issues, family, and school.

Personal Issues

A child's understanding of complex issues is limited by their age. Faulty interpretations can easily be made, and the media offers lots of opportunities for that to happen. For example, someone who caught a near-fatal disease from a cat is interviewed on television. They describe what they did to contract it and then go on to list the symptoms. Sam has been feeling unwell all day (in reality because of three chocolate bars and two fizzy drinks). He sees the interview, thinks he might have done the same with Fluffy, and convinces himself that he also has the symptoms. He starts to worry that he has the same awful disease.

Fears about their health is a common cause for anxiety in children. So too is their sexuality. Without careful, simple explanations of the real facts about diseases, illnesses or sex, it is easy for them to worry about such things and unwittingly create high anxiety levels.

Family

In attempting to bring up children 'correctly', parents can often overlook the need to be supportive even when mistakes are being pointed out or behaviour being corrected. It is far more common for a child to be personally labelled through criticism, rather than the action. For example, a parent may exclaim 'Jo, you stupid thing!' when Jo puts her shoes on the wrong feet. It would be more appropriate (and correct) to say 'Jo, putting shoes on the wrong feet isn't right.' If other negative messages have been given to Jo throughout the day, then she will come to think that she is stupid/silly/careless, because she keeps being told she is. Thus starts the development of poor self-esteem. Parents don't do this deliberately to harm; they may be merely repeating things which their parents said to them when they were young, and are not aware of how damaging those messages can be.

Similarly, in their eagerness to see their child progress, it is easy for parents to expect too much from them and to be over-critical, forgetting that we all need encouragement if we are to learn effectively. Constantly being told that their attempts are inadequate, without equal acknowledgement of what they have achieved, is harmful. Criticism needn't be destructive; it can be constructive, too. If it isn't, children lose their sense of confidence in their own abilities to do anything well. It is important that their need for support is satisfied, even though mistakes are being pointed out.

Feeling inadequate is bound to make any child's anxiety levels rise (or any adult's, for that matter); so too can tensions at home. An argument between the child's parents might lead to worries about mum and dad not getting on and fears about 'what might happen' to the family and to the child itself. Children have very vivid imaginations and it is easy for them to imagine all sorts of awful scenarios, and then worry over what they have imagined. This too can increase anxiety levels and as we know, anxiety can lead to panic attacks.

School

Teachers can make the same mistakes with children as parents: withholding support; putting pressure on to achieve; setting unattainable goals. Peer group pressure can also add to children's anxiety. School should be a joy, but can turn into a nightmare of unbearable misery for some children.

Unfortunately, bullying is common in schools and is another issue which can lead to excessive levels of anxiety in children – understandably. Anybody would be worried if they were in constant danger of being hurt physically or mentally for no apparent reason.

Fear of violence in general and of war in particular is also a common worry in children. Again, this is perhaps the result of misinterpreting snatches of news and conversations without proper understanding of what has been said. These topics are ones which can also easily encourage fears of inability to cope, should the worst happen (the bomb drop/wholesale massacre/etc.) and can easily trigger unwelcome, persistent thoughts.

Identifying actual worries may be difficult. For example, a child who develops school phobia may in fact have worries over getting undressed for gym. Root causes of anxieties may be unknown to the child. You could help to explore them in various ways: through their drawings, paintings or story making. Young children may reveal their anxieties through play activities. Listen carefully to their chatter for clues. They tend to act out problems with toys and through imaginary conversations. Then once you know what is causing the anxiety, you can start to help them do something about it.

What You Can Do

Panic attacks and anxiety in children may serve a useful purpose, in the same way as they do for some adults. It could be that through them they receive the understanding, sympathy and attention which would otherwise be missing in their lives. Because of this there may be some resistance towards attempts to remove the attacks. The threatened loss of loving care might create a much stronger fear than any they have about panic attacks. If this is the case, reassurance will be important, as well as encouragement and support in finding exciting interests and activities which could fill gaps left by the absence of panic attacks.

Prevention is always better than cure, and giving lots of reassurance to children is a sound investment. It will help allay fears and through a renewed sense of security, self-confidence can develop. Self-confidence and anxiety are poor bedfellows.

It will mean giving lots of encouragement. Praising successes will help build their possibly flagging self-esteem, and overhearing you praise them to others is even better. A wrapping-in-cotton-wool approach, to try and secure them against possible unpleasantness, might be understandable but it won't help. Instead, they need to find the courage to explore their own sense of independence, which they can only do with active support from others. They need to feel they can rise to the challenge of manageable levels of responsibility. And when they reach them, they can experience a real sense of achievement. By providing a secure framework and environment for them where they can begin to feel that their attempts will not be ridiculed, their fear of failure will start to recede.

That's not to say that failures won't happen, but how you respond to them is important. Remember that the action should be labelled, not the child. Pointing out how frightened or silly they feel, and mocking those feelings, only serves to diminish their sense of self-worth. Whether we as adults see how ridiculous it is to feel scared in certain situations is unimportant. What is important is acknowledgement of their feelings. There is nothing right or wrong about them. You cannot judge feelings. Feelings are right and true for that person, and if they are unpleasant or distressing ones it needs understanding from others to help alleviate or come to terms with them.

So failures, when they inevitably happen, should be acknowledged but dealt with carefully by you. Listen to what they want to say about it. Don't try to deny either what they feel or the truth of the experience. But do reinforce your care and support for them regardless of their failures and failings. Show them the meaning of unconditional love.

Actively listening to children is something which can be easily overlooked by adults. Your own worries about tomorrow's meeting or tonight's dinner seem far more important to you. However, ignoring children is another way of undermining their self-esteem. The message to them is that they aren't important enough to listen to, and with time they may even stop trying, even though they have important worries. Instead they keep them inside, festering away and eventually transforming into anxiety. Communication is important to children. Without it, how else can they learn; how else can they ask about the things they need to question; how else can they find reassurances about their worries? They need to know they can talk and be heard. Learning to listen more actively could be a very positive way, not only to help them improve their sense of self-worth, but also to provide opportunities for them to reveal anxieties, talk them through and find the support and reassurance which they need from you.

Children are impressionable. They also identify well with role models. This fact can be used to help them in situations which they find difficult and which raise their levels of anxiety. There may be someone in their life whom they particularly admire – it can be a real or fictional character. Or you could invent a character together who has those attributes which they would like to have, e.g. fearlessness or calmness. You could then act out situations with them, suggesting positive things they might do if they were their role model. You could get them to try to imagine how they might think if they were that person, too, if troublesome thoughts are a problem. Try these games as a way of helping them learn new, more positive behaviour patterns.

There may also be practical skills which would be of direct help to them in coping more constructively with situations they find difficult. For example, if examinations prompt anxiety or panic attacks, learning specific study skills could be of real help. If fear of personal violence affects them, then a course in self-defence might help regain a sense of confidence in being able to take care of themselves. By example, you could also show them positive and confident attitudes towards those types of situations which can be stressful e.g. going to new places. If they see you excited but not worried, they may begin to see that they have nothing to fear either.

Apart from these specific suggestions, what has been mentioned in the rest of the book applies here, too. Demystify what panic attacks are, using words appropriate to the child's age. They need to know that they don't have some awful disease which is causing it, and that they aren't peculiar just because none of their friends have the same. Knowing the reason why is important for everyone, including children.

During an Attack

If you are with your child when they have an attack, you can use your presence to help minimize the impact of the sensations they experience. Stay calm; it will only disturb them more if they see you worried or alarmed. You know that the attack will pass, leaving them unharmed, and knowing this should help you stay unruffled. Try to communicate your calmness to them. Holding their hand and saying soothing words may help. Hold them tightly and give them a big hug if you think that might help, and perhaps gently rock them. Physical contact can be very soothing and reassuring.

They may be alarmed at what they are experiencing. Tell them that they are all right and that no harm will come to them, just the same as you would with an adult. Acknowledge how they feel and remind them that it will pass and soon be over. Remind them also of the explanation you gave beforehand of why it is happening. It will help them to understand in the moment what is causing the things they feel. And if they have practised acting like their role model, with your help, you could try reminding them of what that person might do now if it were happening to them. Recall the things you said and did in the games you played together.

As they come out of it, it may help to look with them at what might have triggered the attack. Talking openly about it might provide a good opportunity to discuss their fears and allay some of them through giving lots of immediate reassurances.

If attacks tend to happen when you're not there, you could practise beforehand what they could do on their own. Develop strategies, much akin to those covered in the book already. What might be of additional help to them is practising those role model stances: feeling floppy, feeling calm, being in control, not being frightened. And if you haven't done so already, consider talking to teachers about the attacks and suggest ways in which they might help. Not making a fuss is one way. Suggesting teachers encourage them to stay *in situ* during an attack is another, and if they do have to leave, supporting them in returning to the situation straight away. If you know that holding your child's hand is of particular help, you might like to tell them of that, as well as other strategies you have developed together.

Story Books

Story books can often help children (and adults) investigate difficult situations, emotions or experiences in a safe environment. They can be a positive help in offering additional reassurances. Here is a list of books which may help. You should be able to find them in, or have them ordered through, your local library. It is by no means an exhaustive list and if you would like something more specific, call in at your local branch and ask the librarian if s/he can recommend some suitable titles for you.

Fear of the Dark
    The Owl Who Was Afraid of the Dark; Jill TOMLINSON. (7–9 years)

Can't You Sleep Little Bear? Martin WADDELL. (4–7)

Shyness/Communication
Fiona Finds Her Tongue; Diana HENDRY. (6–9)
Persuading Stick; J R TOWNSEND. (9–12)

Divorce/Separation
It's Not the End of the World; Judy BLUME. (10+)
The Visitors Who Came to Stay; Annalena McAFFEE. (5–8)

Death (Family/pets)
I'll Always Love You; Hans WILHELM. (5–8)
To Hell with Dying; Alice WALKER. (9+)
Badger's Parting Gifts; Susan VARLEY. (5–8)

Bullying
Blubber; Judy BLUME. (10+)

School
The *Kids of Polk Street School* series; Patricia Reilly GIFF. (5–8)
Taller than Before; Bernard ASHLEY. (7–9)
Michael's First Day at School; Alison COLES. (4–7)

Monsters
Monster Bed; Sean WILLIS. (4–7)

Size/Weight
Titch; Pat HUTCHINS. (4–7)
Big Pink; Ann PILLING. (9+)

Multi-Racial
Comfort Herself; Geraldine KAYE. (9+)

Miscellaneous
Different Dragons; Jean LITTLE. (Fear of dogs) (7+)

What Are You Scared Of? Hanne LARSEN. (4–7)
Won't Somebody Play with Me? Steven KELLOGG. (4–7)
Where the Wild Things Are; Maurice SENDAK. (Daring to face fears)
(4–7)
Scaredy-Cat; Ann FINE. (6+)

Judy Blume and Paula Danziger have written a number of books which concentrate on teenage fears and problems.

There is a useful reference book for parents which you might be able to find in your local library. If they don't have it, ask if they could borrow a copy for you from another library, as unfortunately it is now out of print: *I Need a Book: The Parent's Guide to Children's Books for Special Situations* by Tony Bradman, published by Thorsons, 1987.

Summary

◆ Children have panic attacks, too.
◆ Parents can play a vital role in helping to allay fears and build confidence.
◆ Giving reassurance is vitally important.
◆ Develop games (strategies) which can help teach them more positive behaviour patterns.
◆ Use story books to help investigate, confront and resolve fears.

17

Summary

The book has covered a lot of ground, most of which I hope you found interesting, but more importantly, useful. Initially, it may have been a surprise to hear that others' panic attacks have subsided. I know that while you experience them it is difficult to imagine, especially if your doctor is unsupportive and has given you little hope or confidence. But panic attacks do stop, and I hope you find encouragement in that fact itself. You are a special person – every one of us is – but you're no different in this respect, and I personally believe that it is possible for everyone who has panic attacks to also be without them, until researchers can prove otherwise. And that includes you. Know that they will come to an end and that it is you who will do it, because a) no one else can do it for you, and b) you have a vast amount of as yet untapped potential power to help.

You might also have been surprised at how many different thoughts and theories there are about possible causes. It is hardly surprising that your doctor may come across as having less than the full facts. Unfortunately, they are used to thinking of themselves as the fount of all medical knowledge, and some may feel quite uncomfortable realizing that they don't know how to answer the 'why?' of panic attacks. No one knows, conclusively. There appears to be no one identifiable cause. It could be a biological or a psychological reason why they happen – or it could be a combination of both.

This lack of clarity has meant that finding a 'cure' has been difficult. In the main, biologists say take a pill; psychologists say let's look into your past. But splinter groups do appear to be forming and making headway on their own account, such as those in the biological camp looking into organic brain dysfunction, and those in the other considering cognitive therapy. But what I hope you realize now after reading the book is that whatever treatment is used, it is essentially you who will stop them. It is you who has the power to do that, although it may take some time to acknowledge this fully and come to terms with it. Your body is inextricably inter-linked with your mind, and the power of the thoughts which you generate through it are considerable. After all, it is the thoughts which have been partly responsible for cuing you into attacks; now you can use them to help you out instead.

One way in which you can start to exercise this new appreciation of the power you have is to go and talk again with your doctor. Be pro-active this time; not 'patient'. Ask the receptionist for a longer appointment, take along this book and talk through some of your ideas and ask all those other questions you want answered. Do remember though that they're only human, and if they can't tell you, ask for a referral to someone else who can. You have a right to know, but not to be fobbed off with unsatisfactory explanations.

While reading this book you may have decided that you would like help with trying to identify the causes of your own panic attacks. That's something else you could ask your doctor about. S/he should be able to refer you to someone who could help you do just that; but it is your responsibility to ask for that help, just as it's your responsibility to 'cure' yourself; not mine, the doctor's, or anyone or anything else's. This realization might appear daunting at first, but it isn't as bad as it seems: on the contrary, it gives you the freedom to take charge for yourself of your own well-being and success. You no longer have to wait for others to make you well or happy or panic-free. You can start to take action and make it happen on your own account.

To help you, there are lots of available tools. You can acquire as many as you want or need, and include them in your own panic prevention kit. The book has attempted to provide you with lots of suggestions. Although I am personally wary of the benefits of medication, it might be a tool you decide to include. That's fine, so long as you understand the role you want it to play, and that you choose decisively to use it and in full knowledge of the facts. This attitude is positive. Being railroaded by doctors into taking it isn't.

There are other sorts of professional help which you may now decide you would like to form part of your tool kit, such as confidence-building activities and psychotherapy. Study them with discrimination. Weigh up the good and bad points for you, personally. What could be of direct help to one person may be useless to another. You are an individual with your own wants and needs, so choose your own preferences.

However, if you find yourself putting barriers up about all suggestions, and are negative about every potentially helpful comment, you need to ask yourself whether you really want your panic attacks to subside. They may be serving a useful role in your life. Ask yourself what you are scared of facing or losing if the attacks stopped. An honest answer may be difficult to find on your own. A counsellor or psychotherapist's help might support your search. Ask your doctor for a referral if you think this might be the case with you.

Learning to accept your panic attacks fully when they happen might be one of the most difficult strategies mentioned in the book. Hopefully, arming yourself with your new-found knowledge will help make it easier for you. Removing that resistance against acceptance is important. In doing so you help remove the fear.

Use some of the strategies suggested to start developing your own personalized action plan. Be selective about what you choose. They are suggestions – not prescriptions. You don't have to do all of them. Take control, and choose your own selection.

You may want to go back and read some parts of the book a second time to remind yourself of the facts. The more you know, the easier it will be to keep that fear at bay, reassure yourself and to take control.

I hope this book has inspired you and given you the courage to look at *you*, your life, the people in it, and your panic attacks. They are all inter-linked just as your mind and body are. Be brave. Face and accept not only your panic attacks, but also those things in your life which may be contributing factors to them, such as unresolved anxiety-provoking conflicts, difficult personal or professional relationships, and poor lifestyle habits. Learning to master one aspect of your life can have a dramatic effect on others. Assertively re-allocating tasks at home may help relieve the pressure on you, which in turn reduces your anxiety, which may then affect your panic attacks. Excelling in a newly discovered hobby can give you the confidence to tackle potentially panic-provoking situations. I hope you feel encouraged to look at your life and see how you can improve it. Anything which benefits your sense of well-being and health is a plus to be included.

Perhaps the most important thing which I hope the book has stressed is that although you may still experience some more panic attacks, whenever you do you can now remind yourself that you will come to no harm. Yes, they are unpleasant, but they do pass and will not hurt you. It feels like a heart attack, but it isn't. You think you're losing your mind, but you aren't. I hope the book has managed to reassure you about that, and given you the courage to face them more easily and with less fear. The knowledge that they happen because your body is, in effect, trying to keep you safe, by preparing you to fight or take flight, will hopefully bring you some comfort. These thoughts in themselves may bring you a great deal of relief and reduce your anxiety about the possibility of your next attack.

I would like to finish with a quote from Karen. Through her panic attacks she developed a greater insight into herself, her life, her problems. She writes:

'It is best to find your own ways. If you find something that helps, but others don't agree, forget them; it's your life and whatever gets you through the night is the only way. Don't expect overnight recovery – it takes a long time to get there and probably as long to get out! So take your time.

'You're not alone.'

Appendix A:

Further Help and Information

UK ADDRESSES
First Steps to Freedom
Avon Court
School Lane
Kenilworth CV8 2GX
Tel: 01926 864473
Helpline: 01926 851608. The helpline is staffed by trained volunteers from 10am to 10pm, 365 days a year.
Website: www.firststeps.demon.co.uk

Health Information First
Funded by the Health Authorities, this telephone helpline provides information about local support groups as well as further information on a range of health topics.
National Helpline: 0800 665544

Institute for Complementary Medicine
PO Box 194
London SE16 1QZ
Tel: 020 7237 5165
Advice on where to go for further help and information on specific complementary therapies.

Institute for Neuro-Physiological Psychology
Warwick House
4 Stanley Place
Chester CH1 2LU
Tel: 01244 311414
The Institute is a private practice, concerned with Organic Brain
Dysfunction. It takes self-referrals from people who experience
panic attacks and/or agoraphobia.

MIND
MIND has information sheets on stress, anxiety, panic attacks,
tranquillizers and talking treatments. Some local MIND
associations run self-help groups. Contact the address below for
details of your local branch or see your local telephone directory.
Granta House
15–19 Broadway
London E15 4BQ
Tel: 020 8519 2122
Helpline: 0845 766 0163 (Mon-Fri 9.15am – 4.45pm)
Website: www.mind.org.uk

MIND CYMRU
Third Floor
Quebec House
Castlebridge Road East
Cardiff CF11 9AB
Tel: 01222 395123
Website: www.mind.org.uk/cymru

National Phobic Society
Zion CHRC
Royce Road
Hulme
Manchester M15 5FQ
Tel: 0161 227 9898 (Mon-Fri 10.30am – 4pm)
This is a membership only organization. Contact them for further details.
Website: www.phobics-society.org.uk
E-mail: natphob.soc@good.co.uk

NHS Direct
Operated by the National Health Service, it provides advice from qualified personnel on health related issues.
National Helpline: 0845 4647
Website: www.nhsdirect.nhs.uk

No Panic
93 Brands Farm Way
Telford
Shropshire TF3 2JQ
Tel: 01952 590005
Helpline: 01952 590545 (10am – 10pm, 365 days a year, confidential and staffed by trained volunteers)
Infoline: 0800 783 1531 (No Panic provides information on local self-help groups, telephone recovery groups and provides useful lists of books, booklets and tapes.)
Website: www.no-panic.co.uk

Northern Ireland Association for Mental Health
Beacon House
80 University Street
Belfast BT7 1HE
Tel: 028 9032 8474

Patient UK
A website for non-medical people which contains listings on
health-related issues.
Website: www.patient.org.uk

PAX
4 Manorbrook
Blackheath
London SE3 9AW
Tel: 020 8318 5026
Website: www.panicattacks.co.uk
This is a membership only organization. Contact them for further
details.

The Samaritans
46 Marshall Street
London W1V 1LR
Tel: 020 7734 2800
National Helpline: 0845 790 9090
Textphone: 0845 790 9192 (for the deaf, hard of hearing or speech
impaired only)
Website: www.samaritans.org.uk
The Samaritans organization specifically helps the suicidal. They
have local operations set up around the country. Consult your tele-
phone directory for the address and telephone number of your local
branch.

Scottish Association for Mental Health
Cumbria House
15 Carlton Court
Glasgow G5 9JP
Tel: 0141 568 7000
Website: www.samh.org.uk
Email: enquire@samh.uk

Triumph Over Phobia (TOP UK)
PO Box 1831
Bath BA2 4YW
Tel: 01225 330353

Non-UK Addresses
AUSTRALIA
Mental Health Council of Australia
PO Box 174
Deakin West
ACT 2600
Australia
Tel: (02) 6285 3100
Helpline: 131114
Kids Helpline: 1800 551 800
Webiste: www.mhca.com.au
Email: admin@mhca.com.au

CANADA
Canadian Mental Health Association
2160 Yonge Street
3rd Floor
Toronto
Canada M4S 2Z3
Tel: (416) 484 7750
Website: www.cmha.ca

IRELAND
Mental Health Association for Ireland
6 Adelaide Street
Dun Laoghire
County Dublin
Tel: 01 284 1166
Website: www.mensana.org
Email: info@mensana.org

NEW ZEALAND
Mental Health Commission
PO Box 12-479
Thorndon
Wellington
New Zealand
Tel: (04) 474 8900
Email: info@mhc.govt.nz

SOUTH AFRICA
Mental Health Information Centre of South Africa
PO Box 19063
Tygerberg, 7505
South Africa
Tel: +27 21 938 9229
Toll free: 0800 600 411 (Calls can be taken in Afrikaans, Xhosa,
Zulu and English)
Website:
www.sun.ac.za/internat/academic/med/sib/mentalhealth/index.htm

USA
American Psychiatric Association
1400 K Street, NW
Washington DC 20005
Tel: (202) 682 6000
Website: www.psych.org (provides good signposting to other US
organisations)
Email: apa@psych.org

Appendix B:

Further Reading List

Cured to Death: The Effects of Prescription Drugs, Arabella Melville and Colin Johnson (Secker and Warburg, 1982).

What Everyone Should Know About Drugs, Kenneth Leech (Sheldon Press, 1983).

Coming off Tranquillizers and Sleeping Pills, Shirley Trickett (Thorsons, 1991).

Next, Please! Sorry to Bother You, Doctor. It's Me Again, Doctor, Andrew Hamilton (Lion, 1989).

An A–Z of Alternative Medicine, B Hafen and K Frandsen (Sheldon Press, 1984).

The Alternative Health Guide, Brian Inglis and Ruth West (Mermaid Books, 1983).

How to Control Your Drinking, Drs Miller and Munoz (Sheldon Press, 1983).

Don't Say 'Yes' When You Want to Say 'No', Herbert Fensterheim and Jean Baer (Futura, 1987).

Reclaim Your Power: The Secret Art of Maximizing Your Potential, Kaleghl Quinn (Thorsons, 1991).

Your Maximum Mind, Herbert Benson (Aquarian Press, 1988).

Positive Thinking, Vera Peiffer (Element Books, 1989).

Success Through a Positive Mental Attitude, Napoleon Hill and W Clement Stone (Thorsons, 1990).

Think Your Way to Happiness, Dr Windy Dryden and Jack Gordon (Sheldon Press, 1990).

All in the Mind? Think Yourself Better, Dr Brian Roet (Optima, 1987).

Self-Healing: Use Your Mind to Heal Your Body, Louis Proto (Piatkus, 1990).

Matthew Manning's Guide to Self Healing, Matthew Manning (Thorsons, 1989).

Thorsons' Complete Guide to Vitamins and Minerals, Leonard Mervyn (Thorsons, 1989).

The A–Z of Nutritional Health, Adrienne Mayes (Thorsons, 1991).

Nutrition and Mental Health, Dr Carl C Pfeiffer (Thorsons, 1991).

The Health and Fitness Handbook, Ed by Miriam Polunin (Sphere, 1983).

Relaxation and Meditation Techniques, Leon Chaitow (Thorsons, 1984).

Simple Relaxation, Laura Mitchell (John Murray, 1987).

The Relaxation Response, Herbert Benson (Avon, 1976).

Helping Children Cope with Stress, Ursula Markham (Sheldon Press, 1990).

How to Bring Up Your Child Successfully, Dr Paul Hauck (Sheldon Press, 1982).

Helping Your Anxious Child, David Lewis (Methuen, 1988).

How to Solve Your Problems, Brenda Rogers (Sheldon Press, 1991).

Don't Do. Delegate! The Secret Power of Successful Managers, James M Jenkins and John M Kelly (Kogan Page, 1986).

Making Time Work for You: An Inner Guide to Time Management, Marek Gitlin (Sheldon Press, 1990).

Living Alone – A Woman's Guide, Liz McNeill Taylor (Sheldon Press, 1987).

Loneliness, Dr Tony Lake (Sheldon Press, 1986).

The Nervous Person's Companion, Dr Kenneth Hambly (Sheldon Press, 1988).

Banish Anxiety, Dr Kenneth Hambly (Thorsons, 1991).

Peace From Nervous Suffering, Dr Claire Weekes (Angus and Robertson, 1972).

How to Stop Worrying, Frank Tallis (Sheldon Press, 1990).

Simple Effective Treatment for Agoraphobia, Dr Claire Weekes (Bantam, 1979).

How to Stand Up for Yourself, Dr Paul Hauck (Sheldon Press, 1983).

A Woman In Your Own Right, Anne Dickinson (Quartet, 1987).

Making Relationships Work, Christine Sandford and Wyn Beardsley (Sheldon Press, 1985).

Living Through Personal Crisis, Ann Kaiser Stearns (Sheldon Press, 1987).

Smile Therapy, Liz Hodgkinson (Optima, 1987).

Not All in the Mind, Richard Mackarness (Pan, 1980).

Messages – The Communication Skills Book, Matthew McKay, Martha Davis and Patrick Fanning (New Harbinger Publications, USA, 1985).

Making the Most of Yourself, Gill Cox and Sheila Dainow (Sheldon Press, 1986).

Staying OK, Amy and Thomas Harris (Pan, 1986).

Your Erroneous Zones, Dr Wayne D Dyer (Sphere, 1989).

I Want to Change But I Don't Know How, Tom Rusk and Randy Read (Thorsons, 1991).

Beyond Biofeedback, Elmer and Alyce Green (Delacorte Press, USA, 1977).

Cognitive Therapy and the Emotional Disorders, Aaron T Beck (Penguin, 1989).

How to Improve Your Confidence, Dr Kenneth Hambly (Sheldon Press, 1987).

Practical Visualization: Self-Development Through Visualization and Affirmation, Chris Odle (Thorsons, 1991).

Bibliography

Jenni Adams, *Stress: A New Positive Approach* (David and Charles, 1989).

James C Ballenger MD, 'Long-Term Pharmacologic Treatment of Panic Disorder', *Journal of Clinical Psychiatry* 52:2 (supp) Feb 1991, 18–25.

James C Ballenger MD, 'Drug Treatment of Panic Disorder', *Journal of Psychiatric Research* 24 Supp 1, 1990, 25–26.

D H Barlow, 'Long-Term Outcome for Patients with Panic Disorder Treated with Cognitive-Behavioural Therapy', *Journal of Clinical Psychiatry* Dec 1990, 51 (Supp A), 17–23.

Peter Blythe and David McGlown, 'Agoraphobia – Is it Organic?', *World Medicine* July 1982, 57–58.

S J Bradley, 'Panic Disorder in Children and Adolescents: Review with Examples', *Adolescent Psychiatry* Vol 17, 1990, 433–450.

Sydney Brandon, 'Clinical Perspectives', *Journal of Psychiatric Research*, 24 Supp 1, 1990, 31–32.

Sue Breton, *Don't Panic* (Optima, 1990).

Cherie Carter-Scott, *Negaholics* (Century, N York, 1989).

Carlos Castaneda, *The Teachings of Don Juan: A Yaqui Way of Knowledge* (Penguin, 1970).

Norman Cousins, *Anatomy of an Illness* (Bantam, 1987).

Diagnostic and Statistical Manual of Mental Disorders 3rd Edn Revised, (American Psychiatric Association, Washington DC 1987).

E Elomaa and K Aho, 'Toxicity of D-lactate', lett, *Lancet* Vol 336, 945.

Hilary Evans, *Frontiers of Reality* (Aquarian, 1989).

Juan Ramon de la Fuente, 'Efficacy of Acute Treatment in Second Phase of Cross-National Collaborative Study', *Journal of Psychiatric Research* 24 Supp 1, 1990, 42.

M G Gelder, 'Psychological Treatment of Panic Disorder', *Journal of Psychiatric Research* 24 Supp 1, 1990, 23–24.

Donald W Goodwin, *Anxiety* (OUP, N York, 1986).

Iver Hand, 'Panic and Anxiety: Evidence for Efficacy of Behavioural Therapy', *Journal of Psychiatric Research* 24 Supp 1, 1990, 96–97.

Dr Peter Hanson, *The Joy of Stress* (Pan, 1987).

J Hazell and A J Wilkins, 'A Contribution of Fluorescent Lighting to Agoraphobia', *Psychol Med* Aug 1990, 20 (3), 591–596.

George R Heninger and Dennis S Charney, 'Noradrenergic Mechanisms in the Pathogenesis and Treatment of Panic Disorder', *Journal of Psychiatric Research* 24 Supp 1, 1990, 92–93.

D A Katerndahl, 'Factors Associated with Persons with Panic Attacks Seeking Medical Care', *Family Medicine*, Nov/Dec 1990, 22 (6), 462–466.

Donald F Klein, 'The Pathophysiology of Panic Anxiety', *Journal of Clinical Psychiatry* 52:2 (supp) Feb 1991, 10–11.

Gerald L Klerman MD, 'Panic Disorder: Strategies for Long-Term Treatment. Introduction', *Journal of Clinical Psychiatry* 52:2 (supp) Feb 1991, 3–5.

J Daniel Knofsky et al, 'Seasonal Panic Disorder Responsive to Light Therapy', (let), *Lancet* Vol 337, 4 May 1991.

Reinhard Kowalski, *Over the Top* (Winslow Press, 1987).

Tomifusa Kuboki et al, 'Historical Review of Panic Disorder and Clinical Studies in Japan', *Journal of Psychiatric Research* 24 Supp 1, 1990, 70–72.

Martin Landau-North, *For People who Panic* (Anthos Park, 1985).

R J McNally, 'Psychological Approaches to Panic Disorder: A Review', *Psychol Bull* Nov 1990, 108(3), 403–419.

B Milrod and M K Shaer, 'Psychodynamic Treatment of Panic: Three Case Histories', *Hospital and Community Psychiatry* (Washington), 42:3, 1991, 311–312.

Will Parfitt, *Psychosynthesis* (Element Books, 1990).

Dr Chandra Patel, *Complete Guide to Stress Management* (Optima 1989).

A Roy et al, 'Mental Disorders Among Alcoholics', *Arch Gen Psychiatry* May 1991, 48 (5) 423–427.

Peter Roy-Burne MD Ed, *Anxiety: New Findings for the Clinician* (American Psychiatric Press, USA, 1989).

P M Salkovskis et al, 'Treatment of Panic Attacks Using Cognitive Therapy Without Exposure or Breathing Retraining', *Behav Res Ther* 1991, 29(2), 161–166.

Alan F Schatzberg MD et al, 'Decisions for the Clinician in the Treatment of Panic Disorder: When to Treat, Which Treatment to Use, and How Long to Treat', *Journal of Clinical Psychiatry* 52:2 (supp) Feb 1991, 26–33.

D A Sklare et al, 'Dysequilibrium and Audiovestibular Function in Panic Disorder: Symptom Profiles and Test Findings', *American Journal of Otology*, Sep 1990, 338–341.

John A Talbot et al, Eds, *The American Psychiatric Press Textbook of Psychiatry* (American Psychiatric Press, USA, 1988).

Robyn Vines, *Agoraphobia: The Fear of Panic* (Fontana, 1987).

B Vitiello et al, 'Diagnosis of Panic Disorder in Pre-Pubertal Children', *Journal of Amer Acad Child Adolesc Psychiatry*, Sep 1990, 29 (5), 782–784.

Ruth Horst Vose, *Agoraphobia* (Faber, 1981).

Dr Claire Weekes, *More Help For Your Nerves* (Angus and Robertson, 1989).

Dr Claire Weekes, *The Latest Help For Your Nerves* (Angus and Robertson, 1989).

Myrna M Weissman PhD, 'Panic Disorder: Impact on Quality of Life', *Journal of Clinical Psychiatry* 52:2 (supp) Feb 1991, 6–9.

Index